Mediterranean Diet

*The Beginners Guide To Authentic
Mediterranean Cuisine*

(A Practical Guide And Recipes For Weight Loss And Healthy Eating)

Davet Lebrun

Published by Jason Thawne Publishing House

© Davet Lebrun

Mediterranean Diet: The Beginners Guide To Authentic Mediterranean Cuisine

(A Practical Guide And Recipes For Weight Loss And Healthy Eating)

All Rights Reserved

ISBN 978-1-989749-96-8

This document is geared towards providing exact and reliable information in regards to the topic and issue covered. The publication is sold with the idea that the publisher isn't required to render accounting, officially permitted, or otherwise, qualified services. If advice is necessary, legal or even professional, a practiced individual in the profession should be ordered.

- From a Declaration of Principles which was accepted and approved equally by a Committee of the American Bar Association and a Committee of Publishers and Associations.

In no way is it legal to reproduce, duplicate, or even transmit any part of this document in either electronic means or in printed format. Recording of this publication is strictly prohibited and any storage of this document isn't allowed unless with proper written permission from the publisher. All rights reserved.

The information provided herein is stated to be truthful and consistent, in that any liability, in terms of inattention or otherwise, by any usage or abuse of any policies, processes, or directions contained within is the solitary and also utter responsibility of the recipient reader. Under no circumstances will any legal responsibility or blame be held against the publisher for any reparation, damages, or monetary loss due to the information herein, either directly or indirectly.

Respective authors own all copyrights not held by the publisher.

The information herein is offered for just informational purposes solely, and is universal as so. The presentation of the information is without contract or any type of guarantee assurance.

The trademarks that are used are without any consent, and also the publication of the trademark is without permission or backing by the trademark owner. All trademarks and brands within this book are for clarifying purposes only and are the owned by the owners themselves, not affiliated with this document.

TABLE OF CONTENTS

PART 1 1

INTRODUCTION 2

CHAPTER 1: WHAT IS MEDITERRANEAN DIET? 4

OVERVIEW OF ALLOWED FOODS 4
WHERE TO START 9

CHAPTER 2: HEALTH BENEFITS OF MEDITERRANEAN 13

CHAPTER 3: FOODS TO BE SHOP 17

CHAPTER 4: HOW TO LOSE WEIGHT 21

CHAPTER 5: PORTION SIZES 26

CHAPTER 6: OLIVE OIL 28

WHAT ARE POLYPHENOLS AND HOW DO THEY WORK? 28
OLIVE OIL & OMEGA 3 FATTY ACIDS 29
OLIVE OIL – NATURAL CANCER PREVENTION 29
PROTECTION AGAINST FRAGILE, BRITTLE BONES 30
PROTECTION AGAINST DIABETES 30

CHAPTER 7: PRINCIPLES OF MEDITERRANEAN DIET 31

CHAPTER 8: MEDITERRANEAN RECIPES 33

WHOLE ROASTED FISH WITH LEMON AND OREGANO 36

MEDITERRANEAN PASTA SALAD 38

CONFETTI COUSCOUS 40

MEDITERRANEAN TUNA SALAD 41

MEDITERRANEAN VEGGIE BURGER 43

FENNEL SALAD WITH OLIVES, EGGS, AND TUNA 44

STUFFED GRAPE LEAVES	47
FLAT BELLY GREEK CHICKEN	49
APRICOTS WITH YOGURT AND HONEY	52
BAKLAVA	53
GREEK PIZZA	56
LEMON-TURKEY CUTLETS	57
GRILLED LAMB CHOPS WITH MINT	59
MEDITERRANEAN CROSTINI	61
GREEK SALAD SKEWERS	62
TUSCAN TUNA SALAD WRAP	64
CHICKPEA STEW WITH EGGPLANTS, TOMATOES, AND PEPPERS	66
BARLEY RISOTTO WITH MUSHROOMS	68
HOMEMADE HUMMUS	70
MEATBALL SOUVLAKI	72
ROASTED VEGETABLES	75
CONCLUSION:	77
PART 2	78
THE START	79
MY EXPERIENCE	83
MY JOURNEY	85
BREAKFAST (297 CALORIES)	119

A.M. SNACK (47 CALORIES) 121

DINNER (457 CALORIES) 122

CONCLUSION 142

ABOUT THE AUTHOR... 142

Part 1

Introduction

The Mediterranean diet traditionally includes fruits, vegetables, pasta and rice. For example, residents of Greece eat very little red meat and average nine servings a day of antioxidant-rich fruits and vegetables.

Grains in the Mediterranean region are typically whole grain and usually contain very few unhealthy trans fats, and bread is an important part of the diet there. However, throughout the Mediterranean region, bread is eaten plain or dipped in olive oil — not eaten with butter or margarines, which contain saturated or trans fats.

Nuts are another part of a healthy Mediterranean diet. Nuts are high in fat (approximately 80 percent of their calories come from fat), but most of the fat is not saturated. Because nuts are high in calories, they should not be eaten in large amounts — generally no more than a handful a day. Avoid candied or honey-roasted and heavily salted nuts.

There is no one "right" way to do this diet. There are many countries around the

Mediterranean sea and they didn't all eat the same things.

This article describes the diet that was typically prescribed in the studies that showed it to be an effective way of eating.

Consider all of this as a general guideline, not something written in stone. The plan can be adjusted to individual needs and preferences.

A Mediterranean diet incorporates the traditional healthy living habits of people from countries bordering the Mediterranean Sea, including Italy, France, Greece and Spain.

Mediterranean cuisine varies by region and has a range of definitions, but is largely based on vegetables, fruits, nuts, beans, cereal grains, olive oil and fish.

CHAPTER 1: WHAT IS MEDITERRANEAN DIET?

The Mediterranean diet is a healthy eating plan using the typical foods associated with some sections of the Mediterranean region of Europe.

Not only a healthy way of eating, the Mediterranean diet allows for some food items one would not expect would be allowed if one was trying to lose weight, including olive oil and wine (in limited quantities of course).

This healthy way of eating also focuses on portion control in certain food groups to help ensure weight loss and the reduction in the risk of certain diseases including heart disease, cancer, Parkinson's and Alzheimer's disease.

Overview Of Allowed Foods

The Mediterranean diet food ratios are broken down as follows:

Red meat (4 servings monthly).

Eggs, potatoes, olives, nuts (3 servings per week).

Poultry (4 servings per week).

Fish (6 servings per week).

Dairy products (2 servings per day).

Olive oil (2 servings per day)

Fruit (3 servings per day).

Vegetables (6 servings per day).

Cereals, grains, rice and pasta (8 servings per day).

These must be non-refined.

The Mediterranean diet focuses on the following:

You will eat plant based foods including whole grains, legumes, nuts, fruits and vegetables.

You will use olive oil instead of butter and margarine.

You will use herbs and spices to flavor food. Using less saltisgood for your heart and blood pressure.

You will consume much less red meat, instead focusing on fish and poultry.

You will be able to drink red wine in moderation. This is purely a personal choice, if you do not drink alcohol you do not have to for the diet.

Let's look at each aspect in a little more detail.

The importance of whole grains, legumes, nuts, fruit and vegetables

The people of the Mediterranean area in Europe traditionally eat a diet which includes plenty of whole grains, legumes, nuts, fruits and vegetables. In fact, Greeks are known to consume over eight or more servings of fruits and vegetables daily.

The Mediterranean region also produces many varieties of whole grain. These grains are healthy for you as they contain less unhealthy trans-fats which are known to raise the bad cholesterol levels in your blood. Bread in this region is not eaten with butter, but often eaten dry and dipped in olive oil.

The Mediterranean region is also well known for various forms of nuts and they form an extremely important part of the diet in the region. Although nuts are often high in fat, it is a fat that is in fact healthy for you (but must be eaten in moderation, only a handful per day).

Peanuts do not fall into this group and should be avoided.

Pick healthy fats

The Mediterranean diet does not focus on limiting your fat consumption, but it emphasizes choosing fats that are healthier for you. You will not be consuming any trans-fats as these fats are one of the causes of heart disease.

The primary source of fat on the Mediterranean diet is olive oil. Olive trees abound in this region of Europe so it goes without saying that the oil produced from olives would be a favorite of the local people. Olive oil is a monounsaturated fat. This fat is in fact good for your body as it can help lower low-density lipoprotein (LDL) cholesterol levels. Choose "extra virgin" or "virgin" olive oils as they are the least processed form of this oil and they contain high levels of plant compounds which supply antioxidants to your body. These antioxidants help in the prevention of diseases.

Another oil product that can be used is Canola oil. This oil along with some nut types contain linolenic acid (an omega-3 fatty acid) which is also beneficial to your body as they can decrease blood clotting, lower triglycerides and help decrease blood pressure. Try to use olive oil wherever possible however.

The Mediterranean diet is also known for the high consumption of fatty fish including salmon, sardines, herring, trout and mackerel. Again, these are rich in omega-3 fatty acids.

The use of alcohol

Research has shown that alcohol, drunk in moderation, can help reduce heart disease.

The people of the Mediterranean region drink wine every day. If you follow this diet you may drink the following amounts of red wine daily:

5 ounces for woman.

5 ounces for men over 65.

10 ounces for men younger than 65.

Remember this is a personal choice. You do not need to drink alcohol if you choose not to.

Where To Start

Now that you have some basic knowledge of the Mediterranean diet, let's take a closer look at a few steps to get you started.

Your meals should mostly be made up of vegetables, fruit and whole grains. Aim specifically for unprocessed foods. Fruit and vegetables are perfect for snacks as well. Eat whole grain cereal, bread, rice and pasta.

Legumes are a great source of fiber as well as adding variety to your plate. Aim to eat beans, peas, chickpeas, pulses and lentils.

Nuts provide a good source of fiber, protein and healthy fats your body needs. Almonds, cashews, pistachios and walnuts are perfect to add to pasta dishes or to be used as a quick snack when you are busy.

Olive oil is perfect for cooking, using on salads and as a dip for bread. Do not use butter or margarine in your cooking.

Herbs are used extensively in Mediterranean cooking. Experiment with various herbs, they are brilliant for adding flavor to your dishes. They also are perfect to use in place of salt.

Fish should be eaten at least twice per week. Aim for salmon, trout, mackerel, sardines and herring. Do not fry the fish, but rather grill, boil or bake it.

Red meat should only be eaten a few times a month. If you do eat red meat, make sure it is a lean cut and keep portion sizes small. Do not eat processed meats which are high in fat.

Limit your dairy intake to low fat products such as fat-free yoghurt, skim milk and low-fat cheeses.

"I've never been a huge sweets eater, and I've loved a Mediterranean diet. We eat a lot of dark leafy greens and a couple of meals each week are meat-free. We enjoy eating a balanced diet." Rachael Ray, celebrity chef.

"The Mediterranean diet is rich in fruits and vegetables, while low in sodium. It is also enriched with olive oil, high in antioxidants as well as monounsaturated and polyunsaturated fats." – David Perlmutter MD, renowned neurologist.

There are many different diets available today. Choosing the one that will work for you can be very difficult.

The good thing about the Mediterranean diet is that it is not a diet in the modern sense of the word. It is a healthy way of eating taken from natural dietary models of southern Italy, Greece and Spain. Most of the ingredients you will eat on the Mediterranean diet are extremely good for you and have proven benefits. The diet also includes ingredients that have been shown to fight disease and ill health.

Research has shown that the Mediterranean diet can cause:

A reduction in the risk of heart disease.

A reduction in the risk of cancer.

A reduction in the risk of Parkinson's disease.

A reduction in the risk of Alzheimer's disease.

The Mediterranean diet truly is a way of eating you can follow that will not only help you to lose weight, but will keep you healthy and protect you against disease.

CHAPTER 2: HEALTH BENEFITS OF MEDITERRANEAN

Eating this diet, which is rich in fruits and vegetables, healthy fats, and whole grains, can lower your risk for certain health problems. In this video, see the seven ways you can improve your health by eating the Mediterranean Diet.

When you think about Mediterranean food, your mind may go to pizza and pasta from Italy, or lamb chops from Greece, but these dishes don't fit into the healthy dietary plans advertised as "Mediterranean." A true Mediterranean diet consists mainly of fruits and vegetables, seafood, olive oil, hearty grains, and other foods that help fight against heart disease, certain cancers, diabetes, and cognitive decline. It's a diet worth chasing; making the switch from pepperoni and pasta to fish and avocados may take some effort, but you could soon be on a path to a healthier and longer life.

We have briefly touched on the health benefits of the Mediterranean diet, but let's look at them a little closer.

Protects against type 2 diabetes

As it is so rich in fiber (from the legumes, fruits and vegetables), digestion in the body is slowed down dramatically. This in turn helps to keep blood sugar readings at fairly constant levels.

Reduction in the chance of heart disease and strokes

As the Mediterranean diet does not include any processed foods, refined food and limits the intake of red meat, the risk of heart disease and strokes is dramatically reduced.

Reduction in the chance of cancer

The Mediterranean diet leads to a reduced risk of cancer because of the high intake of fiber, the consumption of fruit and vegetables and cutting out fatty meat products.

Reduces the risk of Alzheimer's disease

By improving cholesterol and blood sugar levels as well as ensuring good blood vessel health, the Mediterranean diet helps reduce the risk of both Alzheimer's disease and dementia.

Reduces the risk of Parkinson's disease

The Mediterranean diet is very high in antioxidants. Antioxidants prevent oxidative stress in the cells, a damaging process that occurs naturally. This cuts the risk of Parkinson's disease by up to 50%.

Reduces the pain of rheumatoid arthritis

The Mediterranean diet will help ease the pain for sufferers of rheumatoid arthritis.

Longer lifespan

As the Mediterranean diet reduces the risk of heart disease and cancer, the chance of death at any time in a person's life is reduced by 20% when following this diet.

Helps to keep you agile

The Mediterranean diet is extremely high in nutrients which help to reduce the chances of muscle weakness by as much as 70 percent in senior's citizens.

Weight loss benefits

Of course the main reason people go on a diet is to lose weight. By following the Mediterranean diet you will see results in over time. Remember this is a lifestyle change. Stick to the Mediterranean way of eating and exercise regularly your weight will drop.

CHAPTER 3: FOODS TO BE SHOP

There are a number of foods that form and integral part of the Mediterranean diet. These foods have the essential nutrients and health promoting properties that have the amazing health effects the Mediterranean diet gives. When stocking up for your journey into Mediterranean eating, you should fill your fridge and pantry with these ingredients.

Vegetables & Fruit

Vegetables include aubergine, asparagus, broccoli, cabbage, carrots, cauliflower, courgettes, cucumbers, garlic, leeks, lettuce, onions, peppers and spinach.

Fruits include apples, bananas, cherries, figs, grapes, melons, olives, oranges, pears, pineapples, plums, tomatoes. Dried fruit and fruit juice are allowed in moderation.

Tinned fruit and vegetables are allowed, but fresh produce is preferred.

Fruit and vegetables are high in fiber, antioxidants and vitamin C.

Whole grain cereals, pasta and rice

Cereals include those made of barley, corn, oats and wheat. These whole grains can be found in cereal flakes, muesli and different porridges.

Do not forget whole meal pasta, whole meal bread, spaghetti, couscous, and polenta.

Whole grains are high in carbohydrates, fiber, vitamins, minerals and anti-inflammatory agents; they help with bowel movement, lower cholesterol and decrease the risk of heart disease.

Legumes

Legumes include beans, chickpeas, lentils and peas. Legumes are high in fiber, protein, carbohydrates and vitamin B and C; they help to reduce the risk of vascular and heart disease.

White, oily fish and other seafood

There are many types of seafood that one can eat including anchovy, cod, crab, haddock, hake, halibut, herring, lobster, mackerel, mullet, mussels, prawn, pilchards, plaice, salmon, sardines, sea bass, sole, squid, turbot, , trout, tuna, whiting and whitebait. Seafood provides protein, vitamins, minerals, omega 3 fatty acids and vitamin A and D. Some seafood is also rich in calcium.

Mono-unsaturated fats

This is mostly consumed in the form of olive oil, a staple of the Mediterranean diet. These fats are also found in avocados, olives and nuts. They help with the absorption of vitamins into your system. Mono-unsaturated fats also protect against heart disease and can help lower blood pressure. Due to their high calorie content, they should be used in moderation.

Lean white meat

This is mostly consumed in the form of poultry, including chicken and turkey but can include rabbit. It is high in protein, vitamin B12 and minerals.

Nuts

This includes almonds, brazil nuts, chestnuts, cashews and walnuts. Nuts are high in protein, fiber, vitamins and minerals. Nuts help to protect against heart disease and type 2 diabetes. They also help to lower cholesterol levels. Limit to a handful a day due to their high calorie content. Eat nuts in a natural form, avoid the salted variety.

CHAPTER 4: HOW TO LOSE WEIGHT

One of the main reasons anyone would undertake a diet or healthy eating plan is to ultimately lose weight.

The Mediterranean diet, although incorporating high calorie foods (such as olive oil), allows you to lose weight as long as you stick to some basic principles.

Remember, there is no quick fix. You will have to be in it for the long run to see the benefits of the lifestyle. The benefit of this diet is that you are eating so many amazing food types, that you barely feel that you are on a diet.

There are a few important aspects that you need to focus on. Let's look at each of them closely.

Lifestyle change

By following the Mediterranean diet you will not only be focusing on eating the correct foods, but on food portion sizes as well.

Exercise also plays a very important part of making a success of the diet. Remember, quick results never last. You want to lose the weight over a long period and in this way you will keep it off.

You can make this change of lifestyle work by setting yourself goals. These goals must be realistic, practical and very importantly, measurable. You are not going to lose 20 lbs in a week.

Calories, don't count them out!

Weight loss is actually very simple. If your body burns more calories than you consume you will lose weight. Unfortunately, metabolic rate (the rate at which our bodies burn calories) is different for everyone and some people burn calories slower than others. This can also be shaped by age, genetics, gender and a person's fitness level.

So, you may think that all you need to do is drastically reduce calories to reduce weight. This will probably work for a week or two but eventually your body will go into a form of starvation mode and hold onto fat to fuel itself. You do not want this to happen.

The great thing about the Mediterranean diet is that it includes lots of low calorie food options such as vegetables. As you are allowed to eat a lot of these low calorie foods, they will help to make you feel more full and satisfied. High calorie food types such as red meats are eaten very rarely on the diet.

Portion sizes

You should also watch portion sizes. This is a great way to reduce your calorie intake especially when it comes to your protein intake, such as fish and poultry. A good rule is that your main protein on your plate should be no bigger than the palm of your hand.

Check your fat calorie intake

As the Mediterranean diet uses a lot of olive oil, you should be sure to use it in moderation. Olive oil, although very good for you, is extremely high in calories. Using too much of it (and thereby consuming to many fat calories), can stop your weight loss and in some cases cause you to put on weight.

Increase your physical activity

Any diet would recommend exercise as a boost to weight loss. The Mediterranean diet is no different. Find some form of exercise that you like and try to do it at least 4 to 5 times a week. Exercise also helps strengthen your heart, decrease stress and as you get fitter, it will raise your energy level.

Food types that help suppress your hunger

The Mediterranean diet is filled with food types that are high in fiber as well as helping to make you feel satisfied and full after a meal. If you feel full and satisfied, it is easy to say to no to other bad food options and to just rely on your snacks to help get you through to the next meal.

The Mediterranean diet comprises of many low glycemic foods that help your blood sugar not to spike erratically, which causes you to feel hungry.

Get your food cravings under control

The Mediterranean diet will help to get your food cravings under control. Cravings can occur for physiological or psychological reasons. It is important to try and control these cravings which you can manage by doing the following:

Do not skip meals.

Make sure you eat at least every 5 hours. Snacks are important to regulate your blood sugar levels between meals.

Eat protein with each meal. This helps to slow down your digestion of each meal you eat, keeping you more satisfied for longer.

Eat high fiber foods with each meal. This includes fruits, vegetables, grains, nuts and legumes.

CHAPTER 5: PORTION SIZES

An important part of any diet is the control of portion sizes and the Mediterranean diet is no different in this regard.

Remember, you will in all probability want to eat as little as possible. After all this is how we have been conditioned to think while we are on diet. If you do this, you are doing more harm than good, because as we have mentioned, your body enters starvation mode and begins to keep the fat to use as fuel.

Good guidelines for Mediterranean diet portion sizes per meal are as follows:

Up to 3 ounces of protein in the form of meat, either chicken, fish or lean pork. You are able to eat red meat but only twice per month.

1 ounce of cheese. No processed cheeses are allowed.

1 medium piece of fruit

1 cup of vegetables

½ cup of grains

Remember to eat a main meal at least every 5 hours and to keep snacks on hand to eat in between meals such as a small fruit, vegetables or nuts (only a handful per day).

CHAPTER 6: OLIVE OIL

As we have learnt, the Mediterranean diet is a very healthy way to eat. It is rich in fiber, omega-3 acids and anti-oxidants which help to stunt or stop many diseases.

Olive oil is actually one of the main providers of these benefits. It contains not only monounsaturated fat (responsible for many health benefits) but recent research has indicated that the polyphenols in the oil also have benefits. These polyphenols have been known to boost the healthy affectsof the Mediterranean diet for those following it.

What Are Polyphenols And How Do They Work?

What exactly are polyphenols? These are antioxidants found in olive oil that help to fight diseases related mostly to aging, including heart disease, high blood pressure, cholesterol and cancer.

One of the main benefits of polyphenols is that they help to increase the high-density lipoprotein levels (or good cholesterol) in the blood. They also reduce triglycerides and low-density lipoprotein (or bad cholesterol).

Olive Oil & Omega 3 Fatty Acids

Omega 3 fatty acids, found in fish and seafood and eaten in abundance on the Mediterranean diet, have many anti-inflammatory benefits as well as offering protection from heart problems. Recent studies have shown that when used in conjunction with olive oil these benefits are increased.

This combination can help reduce atherosclerosis, a disease commonly found in the arteries where fatty material is deposited on the artery wall, which in turn hardens and narrows them, making it more difficult for blood to pass through those areas. This can lead to heart attacks or strokes.

Olive Oil – Natural Cancer Prevention

Various studies worldwide have shown that olive oil can help to prevent the growth of various forms of cancer cells.

The rate of cancer in areas where the Mediterranean diet is followed are much lower than cancer rates in the USA, UK and other countries especially cancers of the bowel, breast and prostate. These cancers are often connected to diet.

Protection Against Fragile, Brittle Bones

Although there is still ongoing research regarding this, the polyphenols in olive oil have shown some significant help in protecting against bones becoming fragile and brittle through aging (a condition called osteoporosis).

Protection Against Diabetes

In ongoing research, polyphenols in olive oil may help to slow down and in some cases stop type 2 diabetes progression.

This research has focused on a pancreatic hormone called amylin which regulates blood sugar levels in conjunction with insulin. Often an abnormal form of amylin called toxic peptide aggregate can actually destroy pancreatic cells responsible for insulin production.

The polyphenols in olive oil (specifically oleuropein), if present during the formation of toxic peptide aggregate can actually stop it from destroying those pancreatic cells that produce insulin.

CHAPTER 7: PRINCIPLES OF MEDITERRANEAN DIET

The Mediterranean Diet is not about quick fix superfoods. Nor is it a strict list of what you should not eat. Rather, the Mediterranean Diet is a formula for healthy day-to-day eating over the long term. Here's a quick guide for those who would like to try it:

FIRST: Maximise your intake of vegetables, peas and beans (legumes), fruits and wholegrain cereals.

SECOND: Limit your red meat intake - fish and poultry are healthier substitutes.

THIRD: Where possible, use mono-unsaturated olive oil or rapeseed oil in place of animal fat such as butter or lard.

FOURTH: Limit your intake of highly processed fast foods and ready meals, which may be high in salt and saturated fat.

FIFTH: Eat no more than moderate amounts of dairy products and preferably low-fat ones.

SIX: Do not add salt to your food at the table - there is already plenty in the food.

SEVEN: Snack on fruit, dried fruit and unsalted nuts rather than cakes, crisps and biscuits.

EIGHT: Drink (red) wine during meals but no more than two small glasses per day.

NINE: Water is the best 'non-alcoholic beverage' (as opposed to sugary drinks), although health benefits have also been claimed for various teas and coffee.

CHAPTER 8: MEDITERRANEAN RECIPES

Eggplant and Tomato Pasta Bake

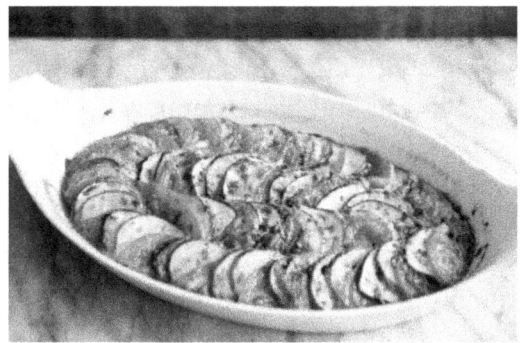

PREP TIME: 15 min
TOTAL TIME: 55 min
SERVINGS: 6

1 lb eggplant, cut into cubes

1 lb sm tomatoes (2" diameter), halved

1 lg red bell pepper, coarsely chopped

1 lg onion, coarsely chopped

8 oz quinoa rotelle (we used Ancient Harvest) or whole wheat fusilli

¼ c basil pesto

4 Tbsp chopped fresh basil

¼ c finely grated Parmesan

1. HEAT broiler. Arrange eggplant, tomatoes (cut side up), bell pepper, and onion on large baking sheet coated with olive oil spray. Coat vegetables with olive oil spray and season with ¼ tsp each salt and black pepper. Broil, stirring vegetables (except tomatoes) halfway through cooking, until tomatoes are slightly charred and giving up their juices and remaining vegetables are golden brown and tender, about 6 minutes for tomatoes and 18 minutes for eggplant, bell pepper, and onion.

2. HEAT oven to 375°F. Prepare pasta per package directions. Drain and toss in bowl with broiled vegetables, pesto, and 2 Tbsp of the basil. Spoon into shallow baking dish (about 2 qt) and top with cheese.

3. COVER with foil and bake until heated through, 15 to 20 minutes. Sprinkle with remaining 2 Tbsp basil.

Creamy Panini

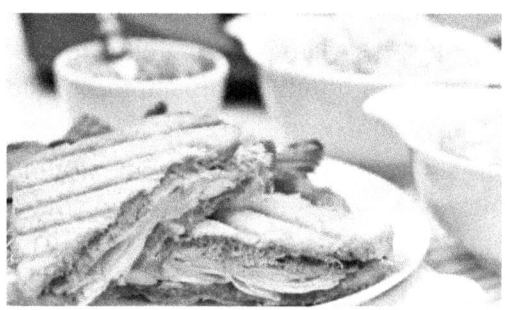

Ingredients

- 1/2 cup Hellmann's® or Best Foods® Mayonnaise Dressing with Olive Oil, divided
- 1/4 cup chopped fresh basil leaves
- 2 tablespoons finely chopped oil-cured black olives
- 8 slices rustic whole grain bread (about 1/2-inch thick)
- 1 small zucchini, thinly sliced
- 4 slices provolone cheese
- 1 jar (7 oz.) roasted red peppers, drained and sliced

How to Make It

Step 1

Combine 1/4 cup Hellmann's® or Best Foods® Mayonnaise Dressing with Olive Oil, basil with olives in small bowl. Evenly spread bread slices with mayonnaise mixture, then layer 4 bread slices with zucchini, provolone, peppers and bacon. Top with remaining 4 bread slices.

Step 2

Spread remaining Mayonnaise on outside of sandwiches and cook in 12-inch nonstick skillet or grill pan over medium heat, turning once, until sandwiches are golden brown and cheese is melted, about 4 minutes.

Whole Roasted Fish With Lemon And Oregano

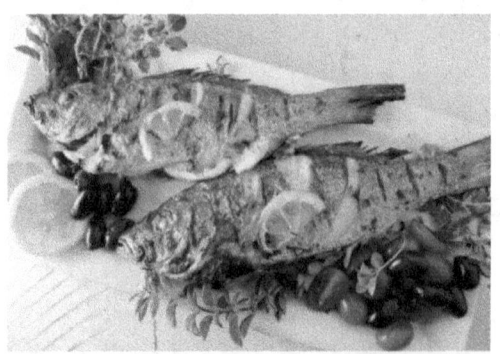

PREP TIME: 20 min
TOTAL TIME: 40 min
SERVINGS: 4

1 Tbsp extra virgin olive oil

2 tsp freshly squeezed lemon juice

½ tsp dried oregano

¼ tsp freshly ground black pepper

1 tsp kosher salt, divided

2 whole sea bass (1¼ lb each), cleaned

2 cloves garlic, sliced

8 thin slices lemon

1. PREHEAT grill or broiler to medium high and coat rack lightly with cooking spray.

2. WHISK together oil, lemon juice, oregano, pepper, and ½ teaspoon of the salt in small bowl. Set aside. Make 3 shallow vertical slits along each side of fish and rub with remaining ½ teaspoon salt. Brush inside of fish with oil mixture and stuff with garlic and lemon slices.

3. GRILL fish 16 to 20 minutes, turning and basting twice with remaining oil mixture, until

fish is golden brown and flesh begins to turn opaque. Let fish rest 10 minutes before serving.

NUTRITION (per serving) 237 cal, 38 g pro, 2 g carbs, 8 g fat, 2 g sat fat, 1 g fiber, 621 mg sodium

Mediterranean Pasta Salad

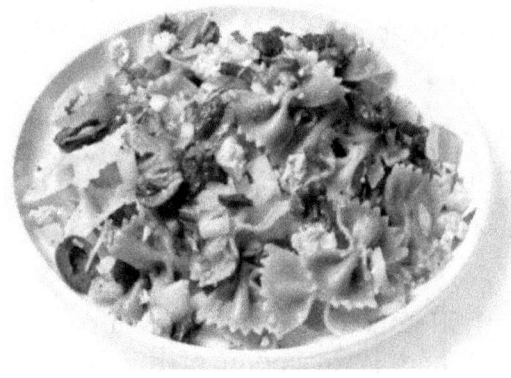

Ingredients
- 8 ounces multigrain farfalle
- Zest and juice of 1 lemon

- 2 teaspoons olive oil
- 1 13.5- ounce can artichoke hearts packed in water, drained and chopped
- 8 ounces fresh part-skim mozzarella cheese, chopped
- 1/4 cup chopped bottled roasted red bell pepper
- 1/4 cup chopped fresh parsley
- 1/2 cup frozen peas

How to Make It

Step 1

Cook pasta according to package instructions, omitting salt and fat.

<u>Step 2</u>

While pasta cooks, combine zest and juice of 1 lemon and 2 teaspoons olive oil in a large bowl; stir well with a whisk. Add artichoke hearts, cheese, bell pepper, and parsley; toss to combine.

Confetti Couscous

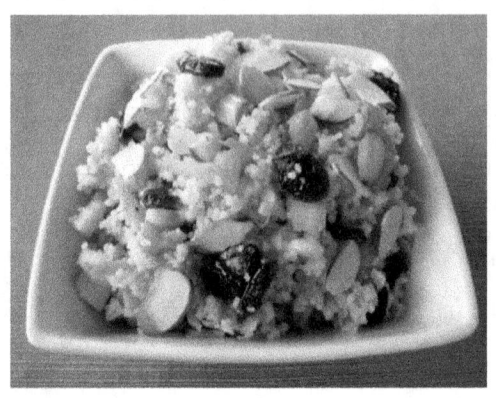

PREP TIME: 8 min
TOTAL TIME: 18 min
SERVINGS: 4

2 c low-sodium chicken or vegetable broth
1 c whole wheat couscous
2 Tbsp golden raisins
2 tsp ground cumin
½ tsp salt
¼ c slivered almonds
¼ c finely chopped red bell pepper
2 Tbsp dried cranberries

¼ c sliced scallions

¼ c chopped dried apricots

3 Tbsp chopped fresh mint

2 Tbsp olive oil

1 Tbsp fresh lemon juice

1 Tbsp finely chopped fresh ginger

1 clove garlic, minced

1. BRING broth to a gentle boil in saucepan over medium heat. Stir in couscous, raisins, cumin, and salt. Cover and remove from heat. Let stand 5 minutes, or until couscous is soft. Uncover, fluff with fork, and let cool 10 minutes.

2. COOK almonds in skillet over medium heat 3 to 5 minutes, or until lightly toasted.

3. STIR almonds, bell pepper, cranberries, scallions, apricots, mint, oil, lemon juice, ginger, and garlic into couscous.

Mediterranean Tuna Salad

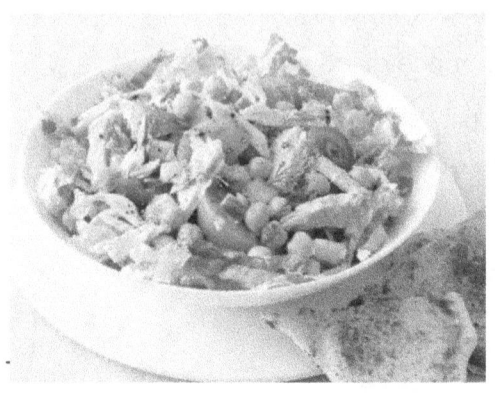

Ingredients

- 2 cans (6 oz. ea.) tuna, drained and flaked
- 1/4 cup Hellmann's® or Best Foods® Mayonnaise Dressing with Olive Oil
- 1/4 cup chopped pitted ripe olives
- 1/4 cup drained and chopped roasted red peppers
- 2 green onions, sliced
- 1 tablespoon small capers, rinsed and drained
- 6 slices whole wheat bread

How to Make It

Step 1

Combine all ingredients except bread in medium bowl. Arrange, if desired, on greens and serve with bread.

Mediterranean Veggie Burger

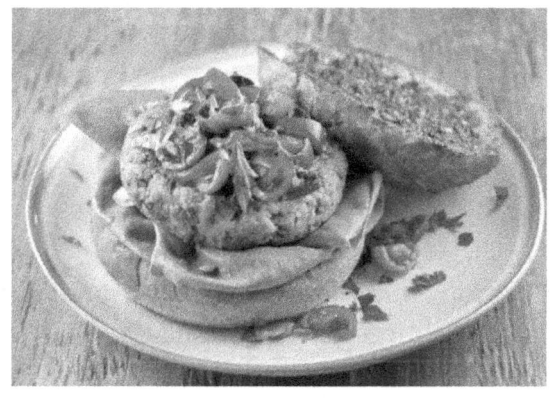

PREP TIME: 15 min

TOTAL TIME: 18 min

SERVINGS: 2

2 lg red leaf lettuce leaves

2 grilled-vegetable soy burgers

2 Tbsp goat cheese

1 bottled roasted red pepper, halved

½ c broccosprouts

½ c baby spinach leaves

1. PLACE the lettuce leaves onto a work surface, with the long sides facing you. With your fingers, press lightly to flatten the center of each.

2. PREPARE the burgers per the package directions for the microwave. Place one on the center of each lettuce leaf. Top each with 1 tablespoon of the cheese, ½ red pepper, and ¼ cup each of the sprouts and spinach. Fold up the bottom and sides of each lettuce leaf to enclose the burgers. Serve immediately.

Fennel Salad With Olives, Eggs, And Tuna

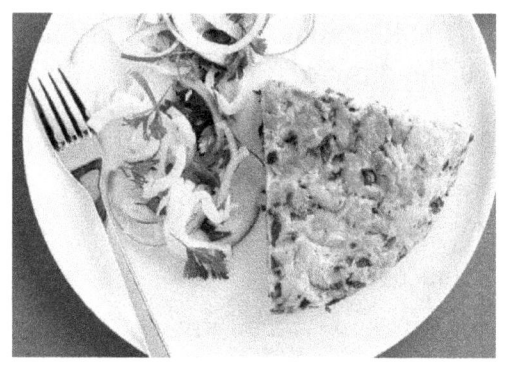

TOTAL TIME: 12 min

Dressing

1 tsp lemon zest

1 Tbsp fresh lemon juice

4 Tbsp olive oil

Salt and freshly ground black pepper

1 tsp chopped fennel greens

Salad

1 sm red onion, peeled and thinly sliced in rounds

White or rice wine vinegar, as needed

1 yellow bell pepper, seeded, veined, and thinly sliced

2 sm fennel bulbs (about ½ lb total, trimmed), thinly sliced lengthwise

8 "French Breakfast" radishes

12 olives, green and black, mixed

2 hard-cooked eggs, quartered

1 sm can tuna, drained

1 Tbsp capers

1. TO MAKE THE DRESSING: In a small bowl, combine the lemon zest, juice, oil, ¼ teaspoon salt and some freshly ground pepper. Whisk vigorously until smooth and well blended. Stir in the fennel greens.

2. TO MAKE THE SALAD: Toss the onion slices in a few tablespoons vinegar and set aside to marinate (turning occasionally so they color brightly) while you assemble the salad. On a large plate, arrange the pepper rings and top with the sliced fennel. Intersperse the radishes (scarlet ends facing outwards) with the olives around the edge. Arrange the hard-cooked eggs attractively in clusters of twos or threes, and mound the tuna in the center. Scatter the capers over the tuna. Drain the onions and set them around or over the salad. Spoon the dressing over all. Add a further pinch or two of salt and pepper, and serve.

Stuffed Grape Leaves

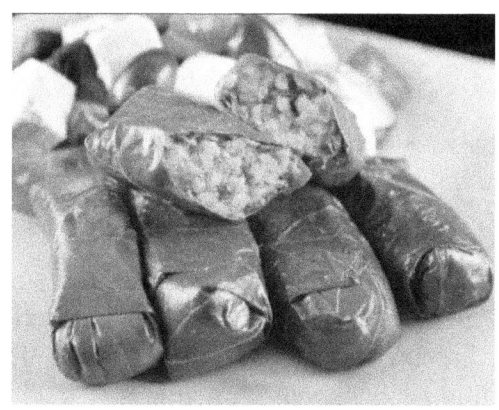

PREP TIME: 20 min
TOTAL TIME: 5 hr 25 min
SERVINGS: 30

1 jar (16 oz) grape leaves, rinsed
1¼ c uncooked short-grain white rice
3½ c de-fatted reduced-sodium chicken broth
5 Tbsp extra-virgin olive oil
1 onion, finely chopped
1 clove garlic, minced
2 Tbsp minced fresh dill
½ c minced fresh parsley

½ c lemon juice

Salt

Ground black pepper

1. USING a knife, remove and discard the stems from the grape leaves. Set aside.

2. IN a medium saucepan, combine the rice and broth. Bring to a boil. Reduce the heat to low, cover and simmer for 20 to 25 minutes, or until the liquid is absorbed. Set aside.

3. IN a medium no-skillet over medium heat, warm 1 tablespoon of the oil. Add the onions and saute for 5 to 8 minutes, or until softened but not browned. Stir in the garlic, dill, parsley and ¼ cup of the lemon juice. Remove from the heat.

4. STIR the onion mixture into the rice. Season with salt and pepper to taste. Set aside.

5. PREHEAT the oven to 350°F.

6. ON a flat surface, place one grape leaf, smooth side down, with the stem end toward you. Using a spoon, place about 1½ tablespoons

of the rice mixture on the leaf 1" from the stem end. Shape the mixture into a cylinder. Fold the stem end over the filling. Roll over once, then fold in the sides and roll up to enclose the filling. Place in a 9" x 13" glass or ceramic baking dish. Repeat with the remaining grape leaves and rice mixture.

7. DRIZZLE the bundles with the remaining 4 tablespoons oil and ¼ cup lemon juice. Cover with foil and bake for 30 minutes.

8. REMOVE from the oven and allow to cool for 10 minutes. Refrigerate for at least 4 hours, basting occasionally with the liquid. Serve chilled.

Recipe Notes: These rice-stuffed grape leaves are best made a day ahead so the flavors have time to blend.

Flat Belly Greek Chicken

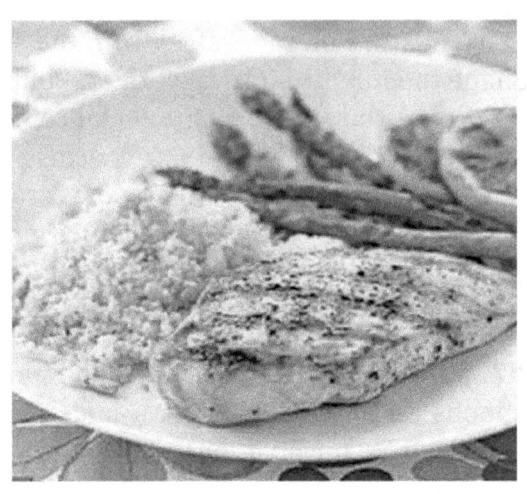

PREP TIME: 2 hr
TOTAL TIME: 2 hr 6 min
SERVINGS: 4

Chicken

4 boneless, skinless chicken breast halves (6 oz each)

1 Tbsp olive oil

1 Tbsp freshly squeezed lemon juice

1 tsp dried oregano 1 clove garlic, minced

½ tsp salt

¼ tsp freshly ground black pepper

Yogurt

1¼ c fat-free greek-style yogurt

½ c shredded cucumber

1 tsp chopped fresh dill

2 cloves garlic, minced

½ c shelled pistachios, coarsely chopped, divided

1. TO PREPARE THE CHICKEN: Place a breast shiny side up with the tip facing you and the thinner side opposite your cutting hand. Place your hand on top of the breast. Hold the knife parallel to the table and carefully insert it into the thickest part of the breast, drawing it almost all the way through. Take care to keep the breast attached on 1 side. Spread the 2 halves as if opening a book and press lightly in the center to flatten. Repeat with the other 3 breast halves.

2. COMBINE the chicken, oil, lemon juice, oregano, and garlic in a bowl and refrigerate for 1 to 2 hours, turning occasionally.

3. TO PREPARE THE YOGURT CHEESE: Meanwhile, place the yogurt in a coffee strainer over a bowl and set in the refrigerator for 1 to 2

hours. Combine the yogurt, cucumber, dill, garlic, and ¼ cup of the pistachios.

4. SET UP the grill for medium-hot directheat grilling. Remove the chicken from the marinade. Sprinkle with the salt and pepper and set on a grill rack that has been coated with oil. Grill for 2 to 3 minutes per side or until the chicken is well marked and cooked through. Place each breast on a serving plate, top with the yogurt cheese, and sprinkle with the remaining ¼ cup pistachios.

Apricots With Yogurt And Honey

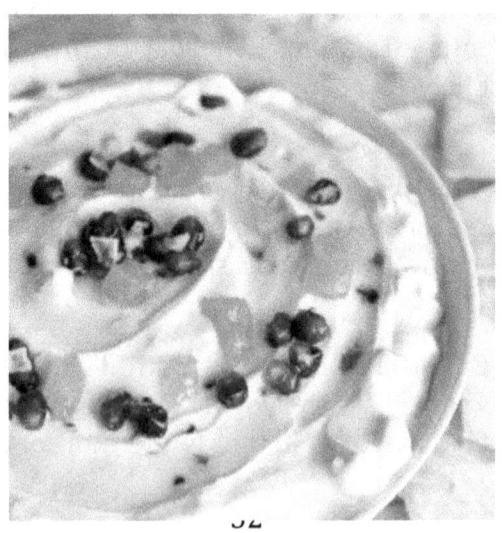

TOTAL TIME: 5 min
SERVINGS: 6

1 c low fat plain Greek style yogurt (we used fage 2%)
2 Tbsp honey
½ tsp vanilla extract
9 fresh apricots, halved lengthwise

Whisk together yogurt, honey, and vanilla extract in small bowl. Spoon over apricots and serve.

Baklava

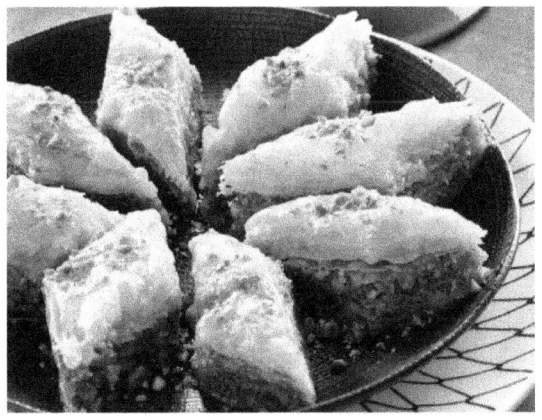

PREP TIME: 15 min
TOTAL TIME: 1 hr 10 min
SERVINGS: 24

3 c unsalted pistachios, coarsely chopped

⅓ c sugar

2 tsp freshly grated orange zest

¼ tsp ground cloves

⅛ tsp salt

Butter-flavored cooking spray

24 sheets (17" x 12" each) frozen phyllo dough, thawed and halved crosswise

1 Tbsp water

¾ c honey

¼ c freshly squeezed orange juice

1 Tbsp freshly squeezed lemon juice

½ tsp ground cardamom

1. PREHEAT the oven to 350°F. Combine the pistachios, sugar, orange zest, cloves, and salt in a medium bowl and set aside.

2. LIGHTLY coat a 9" x 13" baking dish with the cooking spray. Working with 1 phyllo sheet at a

time, place the sheet lengthwise in the bottom of the dish, allowing 1 end to extend over the edges of the dish, and lightly coat with the cooking spray. Repeat the procedure with 5 phyllo sheets and cooking spray for a total of 6 layers. Sprinkle evenly with 1/3 of the reserved nut mixture (about 1 cup). Repeat the procedure with 6 phyllo sheets, cooking spray, and nut mixture 2 more times. Top the last layer of the nut mixture with the remaining 6 phyllo sheets, each lightly coated with cooking spray. Lightly coat the top sheet with cooking spray and press the baklava gently into the dish. Sprinkle the surface with the water.

3. MAKE 4 even lengthwise cuts and 6 even crosswise cuts to form 24 portions, using a sharp knife. Bake for 30 minutes or until the phyllo is golden brown. Remove from the oven.

4. MEANWHILE, combine the honey, orange juice, lemon juice, and cardamom in a medium saucepan over low heat. Cook for 2 minutes or until the honey is completely dissolved.

5. DRIZZLE the honey mixture over the baklava. Place the pan on a rack and cool completely.

Greek Pizza

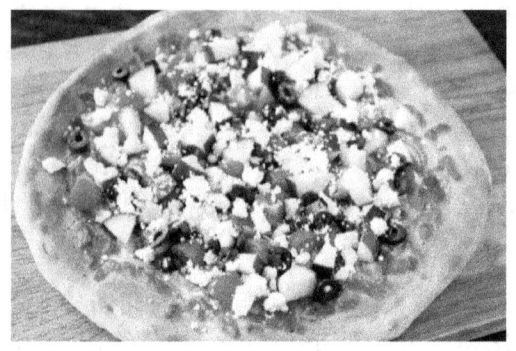

PREP TIME: 5 min
TOTAL TIME: 10 min
SERVINGS: 1

1 slice ready-made pizza crust
2 Tbsp drained roasted red peppers
5 halved grape tomatoes
5 halved pitted kalamata olives
1 Tbsp feta-cheese crumbles

1. TOP pizza crust with peppers, tomatoes, olives, and feta.

2. BAKE in a 375°F oven for 5 to 7 minutes, or until cheese melts.

Lemon-Turkey Cutlets

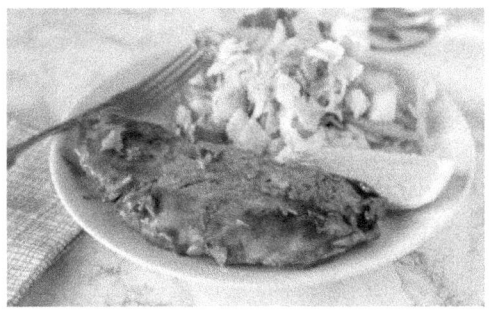

PREP TIME: 10 min
TOTAL TIME: 30 min
SERVINGS: 4

¼ c all-purpose flour
1 lg egg

4 boneless, skinless turkey breast cutlets (1¼ lb total), halved crosswise

2 Tbsp olive oil

8 thin lemon slices (from ½ lemon)

2 Tbsp rinsed and drained capers or pitted green olives, chopped

½ c dry white wine

1 c reduced-sodium chicken broth

1 Tbsp unsalted butter

¼ c chopped flat-leaf parsley (optional)

1. COMBINE flour with 1/4 tsp each salt and pepper on shallow plate. Beat egg with 1 Tbsp water in shallow bowl. Dredge turkey in flour mixture until coated, shaking off excess. Dip in egg mixture to coat, allowing excess to drip off.

2. HEAT oil in large skillet over medium-high heat. Add turkey and cook, turning, until golden brown and almost cooked through, 6 to 7 minutes. Remove to plate.

3. ADD lemon slices and capers to skillet and cook, stirring, until lemon is golden brown, about 2 minutes. Remove lemon to plate. Add wine and then broth and simmer until slightly thickened, about 6 minutes.

4. RETURN turkey to skillet and stir in butter and parsley (if using). Simmer until turkey is cooked through, about 5 minutes longer. Top with lemon slices, if desired.

Grilled Lamb Chops With Mint

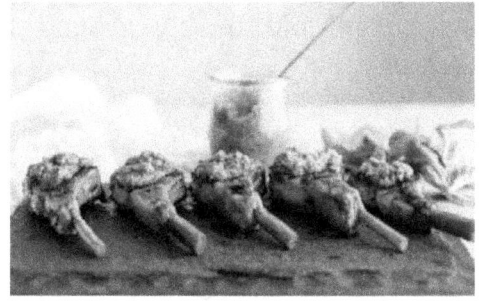

PREP TIME: 10 min
TOTAL TIME: 2 hr 20 min
SERVINGS: 6

1½ c whole milk plain yogurt
1¼ c loosely packed fresh mint leaves

Zest of 1 lemon, freshly grated

Juice of 1 lemon, freshly squeezed

2 Tbsp Michel's spice rub or 1 Tbsp garam masala

½ tsp salt

1½ lb frenched lamb rib chops (about 12), ½" to ¾" thick

1. COMBINE yogurt, mint, lemon zest, lemon juice, and spice powder in food processor or blender. Pulse 2 or 3 times or until blended. Season with salt and freshly ground black pepper to taste.

2. SCOOP half of the yogurt mixture into shallow baking dish. Add lamb and flip to coat both sides. Cover and chill 2 hours, turning once. Reserve remaining yogurt mixture.

3. HEAT grill to medium high. Remove chops from marinade. Discard leftover marinade. Place chops over hottest part of grill and cook about 3 minutes, turning once, or until a thermometer inserted into thickest part registers 140°F.

4. ARRANGE lamb on large warm platter, cover, and let rest 5 minutes. Serve with reserved yogurt sauce.

Mediterranean Crostini

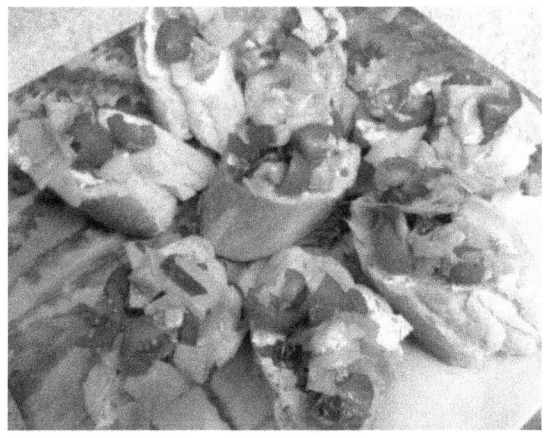

PREP TIME: 15 min
TOTAL TIME: 20 min
SERVINGS: 12

½ clove garlic
Olive oil

Salt

1½ c rinsed and drained white beans

1 c chopped roasted red pepper

¼ c chopped pitted black olives

2 Tbsp olive oil

1 Tbsp lemon juice

1 tsp lemon zest

1 Tbsp drained and rinsed capers

2 Tbsp chopped parsley

¼ tsp freshly ground pepper

1. RUB garlic onto baguettes, then brush lightly with olive oil and sprinkle with salt. Bake at 400°F until lightly toasted, 4 to 5 minutes.

2. MIX beans with pepper, olives, olive oil, lemon juice, lemon zest, capers, parsley, and pepper.

3. TOP toasts with mixture.

Greek Salad Skewers

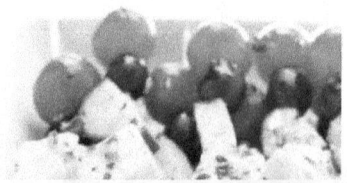

PREP TIME: 20 min
TOTAL TIME: 25 min
SERVINGS: 4

2 oz feta, cubed

2 Tbsp extra virgin olive oil

½ tsp dried oregano

1 lemon, cut into 6 wedges

2 slices (1" thick) Italian bread, cut into 16 cubes (1")

16 cherry tomatoes

1 can (14 oz) artichoke hearts, drained and halved lengthwise

½ sm red onion, cut into 1" cubes

20 inner leaves romaine

1 sm cucumber, sliced

12 assorted pitted olives

1. SOAK 8 bamboo skewers (8"-10") in water 30 minutes.

2. TOSS together feta, oil, and oregano in bowl. Squeeze 2 lemon wedges over top. Season to taste.

3. PREPARE lightly oiled grill for medium heat. Alternately thread bread, tomatoes, artichokes, and onion onto skewers. Coat with olive oil spray and grill, turning carefully, until golden brown (remove before tomatoes begin to fall apart), about 4 minutes. Transfer to plate.

4. ARRANGE lettuce on 4 plates and top each with 2 skewers. Divide cucumber, olives, and feta mixture among plates. Serve with remaining lemon wedges.

Tuscan Tuna Salad Wrap

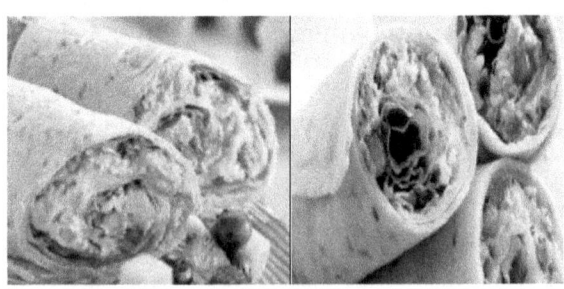

PREP TIME: 20 min
TOTAL TIME: 20 min
SERVINGS: 4

2 Tbsp fat-free Greek-style yogurt

1 Tbsp chopped fresh basil

1 tsp lemon juice

¼ tsp lemon zest

1 can (6 ounces) white tuna packed in water, drained

½ c canned white beans (such as cannellini or great Northern), rinsed and drained

½ c chopped celery

2 Tbsp chopped red onion

4 whole grain omega-3-enriched wraps (8" diameter)

8 tsp prepared tapenade (olive spread)

2 c baby arugula

1. STIR together the yogurt, basil, lemon juice, and lemon zest in a medium bowl. Stir in the tuna, beans, celery, and onion.

2. LAY the wraps on a flat surface and spread each with 1/2 tablespoon of the tapenade. Top with the arugula and tuna mixture. Roll.

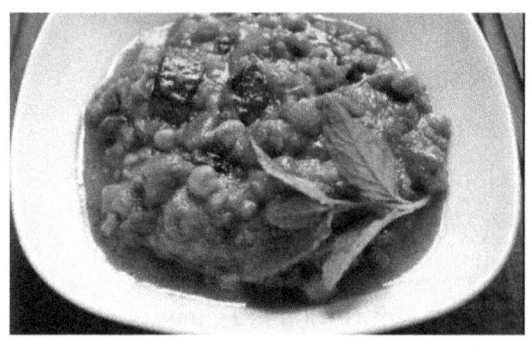

Chickpea Stew with Eggplants, Tomatoes, and Peppers

PREP TIME: 13 min
TOTAL TIME: 1 hr 28 min
SERVINGS: 6

1½ lb eggplant
Salt and freshly ground black pepper, to taste

6 Tbsp olive oil, divided

1 lg onion, diced in 1-inch cubes

1 lg yellow or red bell or other sweet, thick-fleshed pepper, cut into triangles or strips

2 zucchini, cut into rounds 1-2 inches thick

1 tsp paprika

½ tsp turmeric

2 garlic cloves, finely chopped

2 Tbsp tomato paste

½ c or more chunks of tomato, peeled and seeded first, any juices reserved

1 15-oz can chickpeas, preferably organic

8 sprigs cilantro and 8 sprigs parsley, chopped

Harissa, for serving

1. CUT the eggplant into hefty chunks, choosing a shape that works with the variety you have. Sprinkle with salt and pepper and set aside for 30 minutes to release the juices. Rinse quickly and pat dry.

2. HEAT 4 tablespoons of the oil in a wide skillet over high heat until hazy. Add the eggplant and stir quickly. Reduce heat to medium and cook, turning the pieces every few

minutes, until golden, about 10 minutes, then turn off the heat and set aside.

3. WARM the remaining 2 tablespoons oil in a Dutch oven over medium-high heat. Add the onion, pepper pieces, and zucchini and cook until the onions are lightly browned around the edges, 8 to 10 minutes. Toward the end, add the paprika, turmeric, and garlic, taking care not to burn. Stir in the tomato paste, then moisten the pot with a few tablespoons water and scrape up the juices from the bottom. Add the tomatoes, eggplant, chickpeas, 1½ cups water (or the liquid from home-cooked or organic chickpeas), and 1 teaspoon salt. Reduce the heat to a simmer, cover, and cook for 20 minutes, stirring once or twice. Stir in the cilantro and parsley.

Barley Risotto With Mushrooms

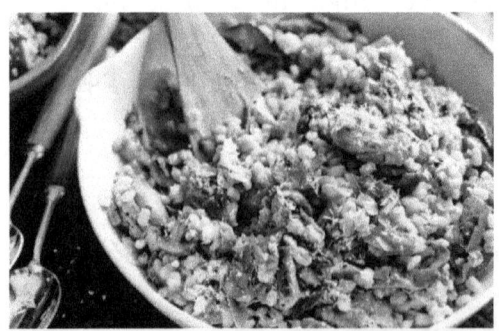

PREP TIME: 15 min
TOTAL TIME: 50 min
SERVINGS: 6

1 oz dried mushrooms

2 c boiling water

2 c fat-free reduced-sodium beef broth

2 tsp olive oil

¼ lb button mushrooms, sliced

1 sm onion, chopped

3 cloves garlic, chopped

1 c barley

2 tsp dried sage

¼ tsp salt

½ c (2 oz) grated Parmesan cheese

1. IN a medium bowl, combine the dried mushrooms and water. Let stand for 15 minutes. Line a fine sieve with a coffee filter or paper towels. Set over a medium saucepan. Pour the mushroom liquid through the sieve. Chop the mushrooms and set aside. Add the

broth to the saucepan. Place over medium-low heat.

2. MEANWHILE, warm the oil in a Dutch oven set over medium heat. Add the button mushrooms, onion, garlic, and reserved dried mushrooms. Cook, stirring occasionally, for 3 to 4 minutes, or until the mushrooms start to soften. Add the barley, sage, and salt. Cook, stirring, for 2 minutes.

3. ADD about 1 cup of the broth mixture. Cook, stirring constantly, for 5 minutes, or until the broth is absorbed. Cook, stirring frequently and adding 1/2 cup of the broth mixture at a time, for 20 to 25 minutes, or until the barley is tender. Top with the Parmesan.

Homemade Hummus

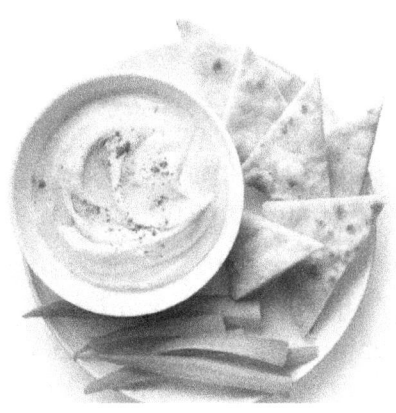

PREP TIME: 10 min
TOTAL TIME: 10 min
SERVINGS: 14

1 can (16 ounces) chick-peas, rinsed and drained

⅓ cup nonfat plain yogurt

¼ cup minced scallions

¼ c packed finely minced fresh parsley

Juice of 2 lemons

5 tsp tahini

1 Tbsp extra-virgin olive oil

3 cloves garlic, minced

⅛ tsp ground black pepper

Reduced-sodium soy sauce

Ground red pepper

1. IN a food processor or blender, process the chick-peas until smooth. Occasionally stop to scrape down the sides of the bowl if necessary.

2. ADD the yogurt, scallions, parsley, lemon juice, tahini, oil, garlic, black pepper and soy sauce. Process until smooth and creamy. (If necessary, add a small amount of water or canned bean liquid to achieve the desired consistency.)

3. TRANSFER to a serving bowl. Sprinkle with the red pepper.

4. SERVE at room temperature with warm wedges of pita bread, whole-grain crackers or crudites.

Meatball Souvlaki

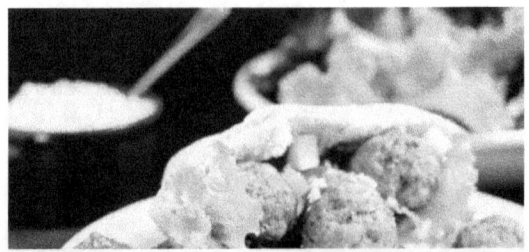

PREP TIME: 25 min
TOTAL TIME: 40 min
SERVINGS: 6

Meatballs
1 egg
¼ c dried bread crumbs
1 tsp dijon mustard
½ tsp dried oregano
¼ tsp salt
¼ tsp ground black pepper
1 lb lean ground beef

Sandwiches
1 c plain low-fat yogurt
½ c grated english cucumber
1 clove garlic, minced
2 Tbsp dried mint
Salt
Ground black pepper
6 pitas, preferably whole wheat
2 c shredded lettuce

2 sm tomatoes, chopped

6 thin slices red onion

1. PREHEAT the oven to 400°F. Line a baking sheet with foil.

2. TO make the meatballs: In a large bowl, whisk together the egg, bread crumbs, mustard, oregano, salt, and pepper. Mix in the ground beef. Shape the mixture into 24 meatballs and place them on the baking sheet. Bake for 15 minutes, or until the meatballs are no longer pink inside.

3. TO assemble the sandwiches: In a small bowl, combine the yogurt, cucumber, garlic, mint, and salt and pepper to taste. Lay the pitas on a clean work surface and spread 1/4 cup of hte yogurt mixture over each.

4. SPRINKLE equal portions of lettuce, tomatoes, and onion over each pita. Top with 4 meatballs each. Fold the pitas in half and serve.

Roasted Vegetables

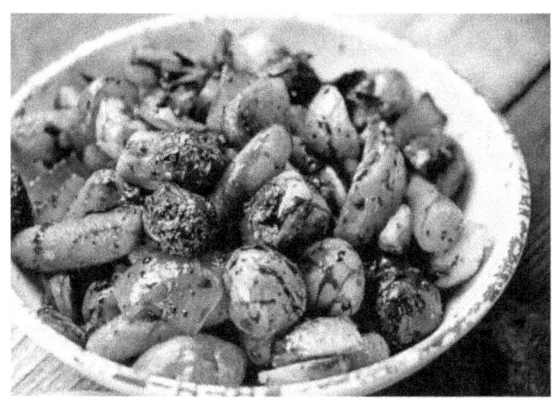

PREP TIME: 15 min
TOTAL TIME: 50 min
SERVINGS: 6

¾ lb carrots, cut into 3-inch pieces

1 lg red bell pepper, cut into ½-inch-wide pieces

1 lg yellow bell pepper, cut into ½-inch-wide pieces

1 red onion, cut into eighths

1 head garlic, divided into unpeeled cloves

2 sprigs fresh rosemary

2 sprigs fresh thyme

5 Tbsp olive oil

Salt and black pepper

2 sm zucchini, cut into 1-inch rounds

2 sm japanese eggplant, unpeeled, cut into 1-inch chunks

1. PREHEAT the oven to 400°F.

2. ON a rimmed baking sheet, toss the carrots, bell peppers, onion, garlic, rosemary, and thyme with 3 tablespoons of the oil. Sprinkle lightly with salt and pepper. Roast for 15 minutes.

3. MEANWHILE, in a small bowl, toss the zucchini and eggplant with the remaining 2 tablespoons oil and sprinkle with salt and pepper.

4. ADD the zucchini and eggplant to the roasting pan and toss. Continue roasting for 20 to 25 minutes, until the vegetables are tender.

5. SQUEEZE the roasted garlic from their skins onto the vegetables and toss well to distribute.

CONCLUSION:

Thank you for purchasing my book.

We hope you have enjoyed this Book and in the process of reading it, learned more about the amazing Mediterranean diet. This healthy way of eating will lead to numerous health benefits for you as well as weight loss over time.

Remember to include exercise in your regime as well to help you get even fitter and healthier.

Part 2

The Start

As a woman, I have always felt the pressure to have to work twice as hard to succeed in many aspects of my life from graduating college with honors and pursuing a dynamic career in advertising to raising a family and having to balance work and family life. I never let my determination waiver and was focused on creating the best life for myself and, eventually, my family. I was focused, ambitious, and felt like no matter how much energy I had already exerted towards reaching my goals, I always had a little bit more to give.

After graduating from college magna cum laude, my determination paid off, and I was the first female to be offered a top position in a prestigious marketing company. This only meant that I would have to work harder to earn the same reputation as my male colleagues, and that's what I did. My sales and advertising record were the best in the company after only two years, and I was on the fast track to promotion.

At thirty years old, I got married to my college sweetheart, bought a house, and began thinking about family planning. However, I was working every day of the week, making sure I had followed up on all leads immediately, my team was on track for deadlines, and every aspect of my department was working the way it should to maintain my record and reputation as one of the leading young marketers.

My typical day began with waking up, guzzling an energy drink, showering, and getting out the door by 6 a.m. On the way to work, I would stop at my favorite fast-food place to grab a large iced coffee and hash browns. I would work all day and was constantly running between clients' offices and my office throughout the day. When 5 o'clock hit, and I had been at the office for 10 hours already, I would relish the quiet and power my way through the stacks of never-ending paperwork and emails.

I would finally leave the office around 6:30 p.m. and be home by 7:30 p.m., grabbing another iced coffee on the way back out to the suburbs my husband and I had moved to after getting married. He usually beat me home and would have dinner ready when I got there.

Dinner in my household consisted of takeout that was put on fine china to resemble a home-cooked meal. All of the food we ate was terrible for us, but it was fast, convenient, and tasted so good. I had gained a few pounds but attributed it to me reaching my thirties and didn't think too much about it because my clothes still fit, mostly, and my husband wasn't complaining. Having a competitive career in marketing, though, meant that those at-home meals with my husband were sometimes few and far between. There were plenty of dinners to be had with partners, clients, and community leaders, which meant even later nights, more calories, and a few alcoholic beverages. By the time I got home, I was ready to hit the sack to start my routine all over again the next day.

Then, one day, we got the surprise of a lifetime—I was 33 years old and pregnant for the first time. My husband was elated and hoped that this meant I would be spending more time at home and less time at the office. He had always wanted me to be a stay-at-home mom, but I had worked too hard and had way too many student loans left to pay off before I could commit to having a family. Yet, there I was, getting ready to embark on an entirely new adventure.

Due to pregnancy complications, I ended up taking a leave of absence from the firm. I was on bedrest or hospitalized for much of my pregnancy and gained much more than the recommended 25 pounds. When you're laying in bed all day, all there is to do is eat, and when you're pregnant at 33, your body just doesn't bounce back from things like that as easily. Because I had retired my corporate wardrobe for yoga pants and t-shirts for the time being, I didn't even realize exactly how much weight I was putting on. The day after my daughter was born, 6 weeks early, I stepped on the scale and had the shock of my life.

After being in decent shape through most of my adult life, I had now ballooned to 200 pounds and barely recognized myself in the mirror. My friends tried to be nice about it, telling me it wasn't my fault, that some people gained more weight than others, and that it was the steroids I had to take that made me get so large. I knew that wasn't it, though. I had lost control. After being so in control of my life for so long, I had used my bedrest and hospitalization as excuses to "take a break," which resulted in me becoming someone I didn't recognize in the mirror.

I couldn't start exercising for 6 weeks after the baby was born, but having a preemie meant even more time needed to be dedicated to her care, and my health took a back seat. One day, while we were trying to take a walk around the block, my knees and ankles started to hurt so bad that I couldn't even make it once around the block. I could barely catch my breath by the time we walked back up the hill to the house. I called my doctor and found out a few days later that my weight was destroying my body very quickly. I had asthma, high cholesterol and blood pressure, and a body weight that was putting too much pressure on my joints and bones.

I began seeing a dietician who encouraged me to look into the Mediterranean diet as a way to eat healthy and lose weight. My eyes were opened to all the ways I had been failing myself health-wise throughout my entire life. I was 35 years old and decided it was now or never. I was determined to live a healthier lifestyle for myself and my family. I knew I would have to give up my iced coffees and takeout and actually learn to cook, but my research lit a spark in me that renewed my ambition and determination and lead me to a whole new goal.

My Experience

12 weeks after my daughter was born, she was cleared to start daycare, and I was ready to get back to work. I had resolved to cut back at work to focus on my family, but now, I also had my health to worry about. I had bought a treadmill for the house, which I was determined to use first thing in the morning before work, and also enrolled in a gym that was close to the daycare. I felt like I was off to a great start, and my husband was excited to partake in the journey with me and signed up for cooking classes. He would prove to be my greatest support system through this journey, and cooking dinner for us every night became a ritual that he savored.

I had many weak moments in the beginning. I had been getting up at 4:30 a.m. to run a mile on the treadmill every morning, which took me about 15 minutes when I first started, and giving up my coffee and morning sugar rush was difficult. I didn't realize how addicted I was to sugar and caffeine until I tried to stop drinking it and it was all I could think about all day. I had to ease my way out of this habit for sure, especially since I had an infant at home. I started drinking coffee without any flavor or sugar and just a splash of almond milk. It took a month for me to give it up completely.

The hardest part of the journey was gaining the discipline back that I needed to conquer the fat. I was tempted every day to stay late at the office, but knowing I had to pick up my daughter from daycare and work out just left no extra time in the day. There were days that I did stay late, asked a family member to pick up my daughter if my husband couldn't get there before close, and skipped my workouts in the evenings to focus on getting my career back on track.

After the first two weeks of going back to work, trying to eat healthy, and jogging in the morning, I stepped on the scale and was shocked to see that I had only lost two pounds. I felt more discouraged than ever and called my dietician. I had to learn the hard way that being fit and healthy required more than just a change in routine; it required an entire lifestyle makeover.

We sat down and developed a detailed meal plan and workout regimen. I began thinking about how I could change my lifestyle to accommodate this new diet. The next day, I informed my superiors that I would only be able to commit to one company dinner per week—only on Fridays—and that I would be lightening my workload to focus on myself and my family. Everyone at the firm completely supported my decisions, and a couple even decided to follow my lead and try out this new healthy lifestyle thing as well!

My Journey

Once I dived into this lifestyle change, I saw results immediately. Sticking to a workout schedule with cardio in the morning and lightweight training in the evening left me with more energy than caffeine ever gave me, and I began to crave and count down to that evening workout. I was eating a healthy breakfast, lunch, and dinner and two snacks—all on the Mediterranean meal plan—and started noticing the pounds melt away. I was also having less stress and anxiety, sleeping better, and had a much more positive demeanor overall. One of the best aspects about the diet was still being able to enjoy the company dinners out but with a glass of red wine and an informed meal decision.

Within just a few weeks, I didn't crave sugar, sweets, or caffeine at all and felt better than I had in my 20s. I no longer had to stay late at the office trying to catch up. My energy throughout the day and positive outlook helped me finish my work quicker, gave me a clearer mind, and gave me even more confidence at work. I was able to keep up my performance at work, and more people were noticing the new me. In just a few weeks, the Mediterranean diet, working out, and other lifestyle changes I had made transformed my life and turned me into a person I didn't even know was there. I started to like what I saw in the mirror, and my marriage improved vastly because we were spending more time together, cooking, working out, and playing with our toddler.

Why the Mediterranean Diet?

The Mediterranean diet is comprised of food that comes from an expansive region including Spain, southern Italy, Greece, Monaco, France, Turkey, and parts of the Middle East. This means that there are nearly endless food choices that make dieting easy, fun, and new. You don't have to put so much focus on what you *can't* have because there are so many foods that you *can* enjoy.

In fact, the staples of Mediterranean food include olives and olive oil, wheat, fresh produce, and wine. Yes, that is right—wine. On this diet, having a glass of red wine with dinner is not only okay but is part of the meal plan! Although, if you are averse to alcohol, you can leave out the red wine and still have all the same great results.

This diet will not only help you to lose weight but will transform the entire way you look at your health and wellness for the better!

Mastering the Mediterranean Diet

The Mediterranean diet was first introduced publicly in 1945 by Doctor Ancel Keys; however, the diet did not begin to catch on in other parts of the world outside of the region until the 1990s. Dr. Keys recognized, while stationed in Italy, that people who follow a diet consistent with this region of the globe have longer life expectancies, fewer deaths from heart disease and stroke, and many other health benefits, including a higher reported quality of life and less stress.

Although Mediterranean cuisine has evolved over the last few centuries as New World foods were introduced in Spain, Greece, France, Italy, and Turkey in the 16th century, the consumption of saturated fats has been the key factor in bettering the health of people in the region. The reduction of saturated fat has directly lead to the lower risk of heart disease and heart attack that people in the Mediterranean have.

Studies of plant-based diets such as the NIH-AARP Diet and Health Study on the Mediterranean diet have concluded that people who follow a largely plant-based diet have beneficial health effects and decreased mortality rates. The Mediterranean diet, although plant-based, is not vegetarian. Fish and chicken are used in many recipes. This diet also has a high salt content as some of the staple food items —olives, salt-cured cheeses, anchovies, and capers—are all high in salt.

Benefits of the Mediterranean Diet

Not only can the Mediterranean Diet help you lose weight fast, but this diet has eight other great health benefits. This makes the Mediterranean diet one of the best all-around diets you could follow.

1. **Promotes strong bones-** JAMA Internal Medicine recently released medical findings that the Mediterranean diet contributes to strong and healthy bones. In a study done by JAMA, participants over the age of 65 who partook in the diet had fewer broken bones and fractures. It was also shown in another study that men retained 80% more calcium while following the Mediterranean diet compared to those who did not. The Mediterranean region also happens to have the lowest risk level for osteoporosis. Many of the foods in the Mediterranean diet are very high in calcium such as cheese, certain berries, pears, and chicken. There is also Vitamin D and potassium, which are also great for combating weak or brittle bones, in high abundance in many recipes for the diet.

2. **Great for Heart Health-** The monounsaturated fat in olive oil, which is used in nearly every recipe, has been proven to be effective at reducing the risk of heart disease or attack. Not only is the olive oil great for your heart, but the main protein staple, fish, is rich in omega-3. Science has shown us that consuming fish three times per week can reduce your risk of heart disease by nearly one third and heart attack by almost 50%. If you suffer from high blood pressure, the Mediterranean diet has been proven by the Warwick Medical School to help reduce blood pressure. Your cholesterol is also protected because the diet restricts red meat, saturated fats, sugar, and butter.

3. **Low in Processed Sugars-** Ideally, ingredients used in the Mediterranean diet will be locally sourced and organic. Understandably, some of the ingredients, like fresh olives, may be hard to find at your local farmer's market depending on where you live. Because all the ingredients should be organic, there will be no high-fructose corn syrup, added sugars, or unrefined cereal products. Typical Western diets consist of many foods that are high in sugar, added sugar especially. When people consume high amounts of glucose, it is turned into fat instead of fuel for our bodies,

which is detrimental to your overall well-being. Although carbohydrates are an important part of our diets for energy production, the Mediterranean diet seeks to find these good carbs in veggies instead of bread.

4. **Cancer Fighter-** Because the Mediterranean diet is plant-based, there are many foods in this diet that are high in antioxidants, fiber, and polyphenols, which are all cancer-fighting agents. Foods such as leafy, green veggies, tomatoes, berries, nuts, and citrus fruits can all help your body combat cancer by protecting your DNA, preventing the growth of mutated cells and slowing tumor growth. In fact, olive oil has been specifically linked to combating colon and bowel cancer. One seasoning and flavor profile that is used frequently in the Mediterranean diet is garlic. This ingredient contains sulfur compounds that seek out and kill cancer cells, slow cell growth, and can stop cancer from forming completely. Other foods that have been known to be beneficial to fighting cancer are whole grains, onions, leeks, and cloves.

5. **Improves Mood Stability-** Red meat as well as greasy and fast food have all been proven to put people who eat them frequently in a bad mood. However, studies

have shown that people with a diet that consists of mostly fruits, vegetables, legumes, nuts, and olive oil are in better moods for longer and are happier overall. This is mostly due to omega 3 fatty acids, which keep the levels of BNDF, which leads to mental disorders, in balance. People who follow the Mediterranean diet have lower instances of depression, anxiety, and mood disorders across all genders. Some of the other foods in the Mediterranean diet that help with mood are fish, especially salmon, and spinach.

6. **Cognitive Health and Development-** The Mediterranean diet has been a part of studies that have concluded that this diet can help battle Parkinson's disease, Alzheimer's, and other types of memory loss and dementia. Some of the most popular ingredients in Mediterranean dishes that promote cognitive health are berries, tomatoes, spinach, kale, cherries, sardines, and other fish that contain omega 3 and 6. These two fatty acids, combined with the anti-inflammatory properties of these foods, are essential for sustaining memory function.

7. **Slow the Signs of Aging-** The primary marker to the signs of aging is a protein called C-reactive, which is inflammatory.

The Mediterranean diet is high in leafy, green veggies that contain anti-inflammatory agents that reduce the amount of C-reactive proteins in your body. Kale and spinach are the two best ingredients in the diet for anti-aging benefits. Because this diet promotes an overall healthy lifestyle, positive attitude, and losing weight to keep it off, people who have lost weight while on the diet and have stayed on the diet can greatly slow down the aging process because excess weight will make you age faster. Berries are great for minimizing wrinkles and helping your skin stay firm with great elasticity. Omega 3 acids are great for skin and hair to shine and grow.

8. **Decrease Risk of Stroke-** Veggie-based diets such as the Mediterranean diet are rich in antioxidants, and also, combining fish, fruit, unrefined grains, legumes, and nuts can greatly lower your risk for having a stroke if you already suffer from heart disease or have had a heart attack. Broccoli is one of the best green vegetables you can include in your recipes and meals that not only reduces your risk of stroke but is very low-calorie and high-fiber, which is very beneficial for weight loss.

The Mediterranean Food Pyramid

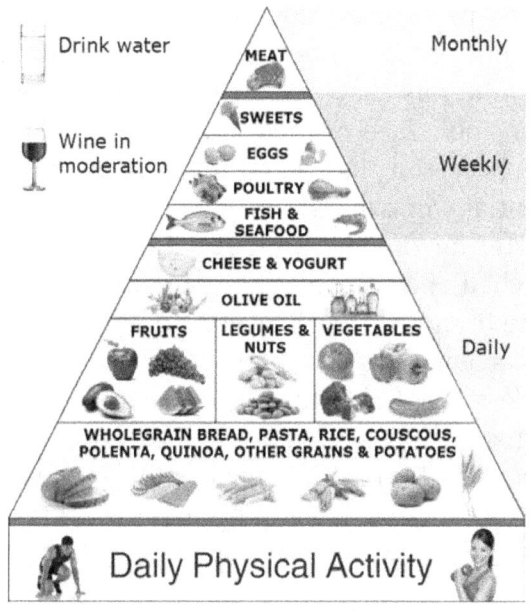

The Mediterranean diet food pyramid starts with a base of daily physical activity. Although the diet can help you lose weight and be healthier on its own, you're going to need to be up and moving every day, whether it be taking a walk, going to the gym, or chasing your toddler at the park. Some sort of daily physical activity is essential to this lifestyle and only further benefits the goals of weight loss, heart health, and bone health.

The pyramid is divided into foods that you should eat daily, weekly, and monthly or occasionally only. The first section of the food pyramid is non-refined carbohydrates. This section is also in the daily category. Whole grains, pasta, rice, couscous, polenta, quinoa, and pita bread contain dietary fiber, vitamins, and minerals that are essential to our health. When foods are refined, that means that they are processed, which removes many of their essential nutrients, making them wasted calories for our bodies that get turned into fat. Enriched and bleached flour (which is in many of the breads on the grocery store shelf), white rice, sugary, cold cereal, refined pasta, and snack cakes should all be avoided. Eight servings per day is suggested for most people; however, if you are trying to lose weight quickly, you may want to discuss lowering this.

The second tier of the food pyramid is fruit, legumes and nuts, and vegetables. The Mediterranean diet is plant-based, so most of your flavors throughout the day will come from fruits and vegetables. Although carbs are the base of the Mediterranean diet with the highest number of recommended servings, the diet still feels much more fruit and veggie-based because the carbs can be something as simple as a piece of pita bread to go with your meal.

Everyone knows that fruits and vegetables are good for you, but many people forget how beneficial legumes are to the body. Legumes are rich in fiber, which aids digestive health and protects against cancer, diabetes, heart disease, and other chronic illnesses. The vitamins and antioxidants in fruits and vegetables further enhance the health benefits as well. Legumes must be cooked prior to consumption to eliminate any risk of toxins, but the cooking process also adds nutritional value to the legumes. Some of the best veggies to consume are those that are low in starch, including eggplant, cauliflower, and artichokes. You should be aiming for six servings of vegetables or legumes and three servings of fruit daily.

Olives and nuts are also part of this tier and are recommended 3-4 times per week but can be eaten more often as well. A handful of olives or almonds makes a great afternoon snack and can pair well with a small wedge of cheese or fruit as well. You can also sprinkle shaved almonds on top of salads for texture. Chestnuts, walnuts, cashews, and seeds are also very good for you. Try sunflower or pumpkin seeds, which provide lots of fiber, vitamins, minerals, and proteins. You should avoid salted or sugared nuts, however, as these can lead to high blood pressure and contribute to obesity.

The third daily tier is olive oil. The health benefits of olive oil have been thoroughly researched, and it has been proven that consuming at least 2 tablespoons of olive oil per day can greatly reduce your risk of heart disease, promote cognitive health, aid in digestion, add shine to your hair, promote healthy skin and nails, and much more. You can easily add olive oil into your diet by using it to dress salads and using it in your cooking preparations in place of butter and vegetable oil.

The fourth and final daily tier is cheese and yogurt. Goat cheese and Greek yogurt are two of the most frequently used dairy ingredients in the Mediterranean. You should be consuming two servings of dairy every day on the Mediterranean diet. Greek yogurt is an excellent source of protein as well as many vitamins and minerals. It is also easy to incorporate into breakfast or as a sour cream substitute. Many dairy products are high in saturated fats, so make sure that you are checking the nutritional labels on the cheeses you are choosing. Sticking to feta, mozzarella, and goat cheese is a way to play it safe. Also, if you don't already drink skim milk, you should switch to it rather than whole milk.

The next section of the pyramid is foods that you should consume weekly. This means that you may not have these foods every day, and that is okay. Much of the Mediterranean diet is plant-based, so there may be some days during the week where you are eating a mostly vegetarian diet. The only meats that are typically used in Mediterranean dishes are seafood and chicken. You may also see some goat used in certain regions as well, but for the purposes of this book, we are going to focus on fish and chicken. Red meats and pork are very sparsely used and should be consumed rarely (they are at the very top of the pyramid).

The first tier of the weekly section is fish. You should have fish six times per week. This means that you should try to use seafood in one of your meals every day of the week but one. If you are someone who doesn't typically find yourself eating a lot of seafood, or you think you don't like it, the Mediterranean diet will be great for you to try seafood in a new way through varied cooking preparations and flavor profiles. Some of the best sources of protein that are also low in fat include fish like cod, halibut, haddock, hake, and plaice. Oily fish such as tuna, salmon, shark, and swordfish are high in omega-3 fatty acids and several vitamins that all help to reduce your risk of heart disease and cancer as well as dementia. There have also been studies linking a high fish diet to lower rates of depression, anxiety, and stress. If you are pregnant or nursing, make sure to consult with your doctor about the best kind of fish for your diet.

The next tier is poultry with a recommended allotment of 4–5 servings per week. You should always remove the skin and trim off any fat that you see before cooking. You can also eat turkey and other lean white meat in the Mediterranean diet. These meats are packed with proteins and lower in animal fat than beef and pork.

The next tier is eggs, which are only recommended three times per week. Eggs are extremely good for you; however, their yolks are very high in cholesterol. If you want to have eggs more than three times per week, opt to use just egg whites instead so that you can cut out the cholesterol. Keep in mind also that if you are baking, the eggs that you use in these dishes count towards your weekly recommended servings.

The last section of the weekly tier is sweets. People in the Mediterranean love to eat socially, and many times, that can mean having dessert. We all know that sugar is bad for you, though, so if you are going to eat sweets, don't eat them more than three times per week and in small portions. Many people use honey as a sweetener in desserts in the Mediterranean. Almond cookies are a favorite amongst many, and using fruit in desserts is popular as well.

Baked apples with honey and cinnamon is a great substitute for pie. You can also make cheesecake with ricotta cheese rather than cream cheese for a healthier dairy option with less fat.

The very top of the tier is red meat. This is the only category for foods that should be eaten rarely or monthly. Save the prime rib for special occasions. Red meat like lamb, beef, and pork has a ton of protein in it, sure, but these foods also have a very high saturated fat content, which leads directly to obesity, high cholesterol, heart disease, and other chronic illnesses. There are super tasty Mediterranean recipes such as lamb stew that are great for special occasions and pack in lots of vegetables.

When it comes to your beverage choices, the Mediterranean diet offers two main options—water or red wine. Everyone should drink at least eight glasses of water per day for proper hydration. If you are especially active, you should drink even more than this on a daily basis. Red wine is the only alcohol that is part of the Mediterranean diet.

Tips and Tricks

If you haven't looked at any recipes yet, you may be overwhelmed with how you are going to fit in all these different foods and prepare your meals to get the recommended servings. When I first began this journey, I didn't know how to cook much of anything besides ramen, so meal prepping and planning was my biggest struggle. Lucky for me, I had a husband who developed a love of cooking and enjoyed preparing dinners. I did learn some tips and tricks along the way, though, that have helped me to actually enjoy planning weekly meal plans and going shopping for new foods.

1. **Curb Your Sweet Tooth with Fruit-** I was a sugar junkie before starting the Mediterranean diet. I couldn't go a morning without an iced coffee with tons of sugar, and I loved cakes, cookies, and brownies just like most people. I almost never bought fruit because it would go bad before I could eat it, so adding fruit into my everyday routine was difficult. Three servings of fruit per day meant having fruit with every meal. Breakfast was as simple as adding a handful of berries to oatmeal. You can also use cranberries, figs, strawberries, and cherries in salads or eat an apple as an afternoon

snack. Fruit is also excellent mixed with Greek yogurt. To curb my sweet tooth, I started eating a small handful of blueberries or blackberries, and before I knew it, I was no longer craving sugary-sweet snacks and desserts!

2. **Get Creative with Vegetables-** We all know the stories of how hard it is to get kids to eat vegetables, and some adults are no different. With six servings of veggies and legumes needed per day, it is important to remember that many of the dishes you prepare may have multiple servings of veggies because they may be completely vegetarian dishes. A good way to add more veggies to your diet is through salad. There are endless combinations for salad, and you can pack in tons of leafy greens with kale and spinach salads. Sliced peppers make a great afternoon snack, and so does carrots or other crunchy veggies with Greek yogurt dip.

3. **Balance the Vegetables-** One easy way to make sure that you are getting in all your servings of vegetables is to ensure that at each meal, your plate is balanced with half vegetables. This is generally equal to two servings. There is almost no need to worry about portion control when eating a plant-based diet, so having an entire plate full that

is mostly veggies is great for people who love food and love to eat but want to remain thin and healthy.

4. **Not All Fats Are Created Equal-** The fats you eat are probably the most important component of the Mediterranean diet. The diet is high in fat but *good* fats like mono and polyunsaturated fats. When grocery shopping, you need to pay attention to the labels and avoid foods that contain any saturated fat. Olive oil should replace butter and any other cooking oil in your home.

5. **Don't Let Labels Fool You-** Many food packaging companies will use misleading language on their packaging that will lead you to believe that the food is better for you than it really is. Calling something 100% whole wheat when the ingredient list doesn't reflect the same or pointing out a really great benefit like fiber while having added high-fructose corn syrup can make you believe you are eating healthy when you really are not.

6. **Drink Responsibly-** Although red wine is a staple of the Mediterranean diet, you should avoid all other alcohols and drink wine in moderation. Red wine is best served at dinner, and one glass a day is enough to achieve all of the health benefits. Alcohol is also completely optional and can be left out

entirely in this diet. The same health benefits that are from red wine can also be achieved through fruits and veggies. However, if you are going out for drinks, never drink beer, and try to stick to red wine if the bar has it.

7. **Go Meatless-** The Mediterranean diet is plant-based. Red meat is not recommended except on rare occasions, and even fish and poultry are not called for every day. You can get plenty of protein through vegetables and legumes like beans. Expect some of your days to be vegetarian, and start searching for fun recipes to incorporate this diet into your routine. Plan 1–2 days a week in which you will go meatless so that your family knows what to expect and you can keep to a routine meal plan.

8. **Stock Up on Olive Oil-** Olive oil and extra virgin olive oil can be used in many different ways in the Mediterranean diet. From using it instead of butter when cooking, creating your own dressings and marinades, or just dipping bread in it, the uses for olive oil are endless. With all the amazing health benefits that come with olive oil, you can be sure that this staple ingredient will be used every single day in some way.

The Science Behind the Mediterranean Diet

A study completed in 2008 revealed that Americans who followed the Mediterranean diet, or stuck as close to it as possible, had their risk of death overall reduced by 20%. The study compared 380,000 people who were following the diet to those who were not. This statistic is pretty astounding.

One of the main reasons behind this is because the Mediterranean diet is high fat. Now, this may make you feel like running for the hills and throwing this book to the side, but there are good fats that our bodies need to function and thrive, and *those* are the fats this diet is high in. Mono and polyunsaturated fats that can be found in olive oil, fish, nuts, legumes, vegetables, and whole grains that the Mediterranean diet is abundant in to promote heart and cognitive health, prevent blood clots in arteries, and lower cholesterol levels significantly.

Being a plant-based diet as well, the Mediterranean diet is high in antioxidants, vitamins, minerals, and nutrients that our bodies need to grow and develop. People that have followed a mostly plant-based diet often report higher levels of happiness, lower levels of stress, mood stability, and other positive emotional aspects of their lives. This diet is beneficial for overall health and wellness in every way possible.

Throughout the Mediterranean region, we have seen lower cases of osteoporosis in postmenopausal women, less risk of heart disease and stroke, and better calcium retention in bones. Combine this with the mental and emotional benefits of the Mediterranean diet and you could definitely agree that the quality of life is also significantly better for those who follow this diet.

The Mediterranean Diet Lifestyle

All throughout the Mediterranean region, when people come together, it is usually over a meal. The Mediterranean diet lifestyle involves making some major changes for some people, including having to cook all of your meals from scratch, carefully planning your meals daily, exercising daily, and cutting back on all alcohol except for red wine.

You will be most successful in this diet if your whole family gets involved in the process. Make cooking dinner a family event. When my husband took cooking classes, he was able to come home and teach me a thing or two in the kitchen. Being with your significant other in the kitchen preparing meals, talking about your day, or just listening to music while you prepare food together can be very therapeutic and beneficial to your marriage. Children are never too young to be involved in cooking either. Teaching them healthy habits while they are young can save them from a lifetime of medical problems and obesity. Go grocery shopping and scope Pinterest for recipes together as a family so that everyone is involved and excited for the process of changing their eating and lifestyle habits.

If you are eating out at a restaurant, there are many dishes that you can eat that are featured at most places. A lot more restaurants are offering vegan and vegetarian dishes that would fit in with the Mediterranean diet. Also, nearly any non-fried seafood dish is perfect. Ask the waitress about whole wheat pasta choices or even gluten free pasta options at Italian restaurants to avoid refined carbs. Always pair your entrée with a side of vegetables, such as broccoli or brown rice. The easiest option is probably to eat a salad, but ask for it to be dressed with olive oil instead. If olive oil is not available, a vinaigrette is your next-best option.

When it comes to alcohol, the Mediterranean guide limits all alcohol to red wine only. Red wines that are made from high fiber Tempranillo grapes can reduce cholesterol by 12% in people that already suffer from high cholesterol. Even people with normal cholesterol levels can see a significant drop to their cholesterol by drinking one glass of red wine per day. There are also tons of antioxidants in red wine called polyphenols, which directly lead to heart health by keeping blood vessels open, free of blood clots, and flexible. These antioxidants can also help you get sick less often, bounce back from sickness quicker, and help with cognitive health as well. There is also research that has been done that links red wine to weight loss through piceatannol, a chemical compound that prevents the growth of fat cells by binding to insulin receptors.

The Mediterranean Guide to Eating and Shopping

When you are out shopping, the experience should be easy. Mediterranean recipes use great, simple ingredients and recipes that are not complex to create beautiful and flavorful dishes that are healthy. Most of your shopping should be done in the outside aisles of the grocery store in produce and fresh meats, seafood, and cheeses. You will also need to visit the bread and grain aisles, where you will fine brown rice, couscous, and other whole grains. When at all possible, purchase organic and locally produced ingredients. Many towns have farmer's markets during warmer months, and even select grocery stores may carry meat that is locally sourced.

Salads are going to be one of the staple meals in your household now and are so simple to make. I always stock up on spinach, almond slices, feta or goat cheese, dried cranberries, olives, peppers, onions, tomatoes, and other produce that may look good the day I am shopping. You can even eat salads on this meal that aren't necessarily a Mediterranean flavor, such as cobb salads with some modifications such as no cheddar cheese, oriental salads, and more.

You can also have salads as a large entrée with fish like salmon or shrimp, grilled chicken, or other lean meat added. Some other great ingredients to add to salads include walnuts, radishes, onion, sun-dried tomatoes, figs, avocado, sunflower seeds, flax seeds, and olive oil.

You can also make your carbs more dynamic as well. If you are eating a baked potato, add Greek yogurt rather than sour cream and butter. Garlic mashed potatoes and rosemary potatoes roasted in olive oil are other great examples of how to get your carbs from potatoes. You can also purchase whole grain pasta, brown rice, and couscous. Rice is always delicious with some vegetables added.

In Mediterranean cooking, you are going to use several different marinades and dressings. Olive oil is the most popular and cost-effective, but extra virgin olive oil (EVOO) is the highest quality. Learning how to make my own salad dressings with olive oil was one of my favorite parts of cooking with the Mediterranean diet. Mixing red wine vinegar or balsamic vinegar with EVOO makes for a very flavorful dressing for salads. There are also many recipes for sunflower oil dressing using lemon juice, tomatoes, honey, and various herbs. You can make your dressing sweet or spicy, ensuring that your salad never gets boring or dull.

Oatmeal and fruit make a great breakfast meal, so stock up on these at the grocery store as well. Any fruit you like can be a part of the Mediterranean diet, but berries and pears are especially great for you and can be found in many of the recipes from the region. Another great breakfast option is Greek yogurt with fruit and granola mixed in.

7-Day Diet Plan for Weight Loss

Most people agree that the Mediterranean diet is the best for weight loss because it includes all the healthiest nutrients that are required to be lean, fit, and healthy. Unlike other diet plans, the Mediterranean diet doesn't aim to cut out fat, carbs, or all sugars, which makes the diet easy to follow and maintain. You don't have to feel as though you are denying yourself anything, which can lead to greater temptation, although there are definitely a few foods such as chips, snack cakes, and soda that need to be cut out of your diet completely.

If you are eating for weight loss, there are several different ways you can eat clean over seven days to maximize results.

1. Eating Fruits and Vegetables- Make a simple salad with spinach or kale, colorful sliced sweet peppers, sunflower seeds, dried cranberries, almond slivers, and olives. If you want some cheese, crumbled feta or goat cheese is best, but you can also use fresh mozzarella sprinkled with basil or oregano as well. Salads can be dressed with homemade salad dressing that you can make at the beginning of the week and store

in a mason jar or olive oil decanter for easy access. Mix extra virgin olive oil with lemon juice, red wine vinegar, or balsamic vinegar to taste.

For breakfast, you can easily cook oats with skim milk and add in a handful of berries or your other favorite fruit. For a bit of sweetness, you can add a teaspoon of honey. Greek yogurt with fruit and granola, avocado toast, and breakfast scrambles with egg whites are also great breakfast choices that can help you get your daily doses of fruit and veggies in.

2. Protein- Most of your protein is going to come from legumes and vegetables. Fish should be consumed 5–6 days per week because of the rich omega-3 fatty acids and protein. Fish and chicken should always be chosen over red meats and are best prepared by grilling, baking, poaching, or sautéing. Never fry it, and always remove the skin and fat from chicken.

3. Seeds and Nuts- A handful of almonds makes for a great snack, and seeds and nuts can also be added into any salad or entrée. They are extremely abundant in antioxidants and monounsaturated fats, which help with cholesterol and blood pressure. These should be a part of your diet every single day and should never be

skipped. They also have a ton of protein, so they help with energy and feeling full for longer. Avoid salted or sugared nuts.

4. Legumes- Black, pinto, kidney, white, fava, garbanzo, cannellini, and all the other types of beans out there are low-fat, packed with fiber and minerals, and great for protein. They can be added into soups, served as side dishes, or mashed with herbs to create great flavor. You should be eating beans at a minimum of three times per week. Lentils are another great option for meals.

5. Healthy oil- We have talked about olive oil over and over again, but this ingredient really must be a staple in your pantry for Mediterranean cooking. The health benefits are enough that if you do nothing else with this diet, you should at least switch to extra virgin olive oil so that you can reduce your risk of heart disease and stroke immediately, especially if you have a history of these conditions in your family.

6. Wine- One glass of red wine at dinner can help with weight loss, cardiovascular health, and mental health. Don't drink more than one glass per day at dinner.

Diet Rules

Carbs are the largest portion of the Mediterranean pyramid, but you must know how best to consume them. Good carbohydrates can be found in fruits and vegetables, not just breads and pastas. The diet is also 35% fat, which can scare many people off, but you should keep in mind that these are good fats that your body can transfer directly into energy.

As a rule, you should count calories and try not to exceed 1,400 per day if you are woman trying to lose weight. You also need to know how many calories you are consuming so that you can track that against what you are burning during your workouts.

Switch to non-fat dairy, limit red meat, eggs, and sweets, and focus on a meal plan that you can enjoy and follow for easy success on the Mediterranean diet.

As with all diets and weight-loss goals, you should consult with your dietician, nutritionist, or primary care physician before starting any new program or changing your eating habits. There are many benefits to the Mediterranean diet that have been proven through science and research; however, everybody is different, and to reach your goals effectively, you should be working closely with a healthcare provider.

7-Day Meal Plan

The Mediterranean diet has been tried and proven to reduce weight and lead to a healthier lifestyle. This diet is great for people who love food because it focuses on all the great things you *can* eat instead of making you feel bad about everything you cannot eat anymore. For best results, consult with a physician and follow an exercise plan to really melt the pounds away.

This meal plan is specifically to lose weight and fuel your daily workouts. The following plan is based on a caloric intake of 1,200 per day.

Day 1:

Breakfast (297 calories)
1 Olive OIl, Honey and Zucchini Muffin
Honey and Olive Oil Zucchini Muffins
Serves: 15-16 regular sized muffins

Ingredients

- 3 cups grated zucchini (I used about 2 whole zucchini)
- 2 beaten eggs
- 2 teaspoons vanilla

- 1 cup olive oil (light or mild tasting)
- ⅔ cup real maple syrup
- ⅓ cup raw honey, softened
- 1½ cups whole wheat flour
- 1½ cups all purpose flour
- 2 teaspoons baking soda
- 2 teaspoons baking powder
- ½ teaspoon salt
- 1½ teaspoons cinnamon

Instructions

1. Preheat the oven to 350 degrees. In a mixing bowl, combine the zucchini, eggs, vanilla, olive oil, maple syrup, and honey. Stir gently until mixed; set aside.

2. In a large mixing bowl, combine the flours, baking soda, baking powder, salt, and cinnamon. Stir to combine and make a well in the middle. Pour the wet mixture from step one into the well and stir just a few times until barely combined. Overmixing makes the muffins tough and hard, so I try to limit myself to 15 big around-the-bowl stirs.

3. Pour the batter in a muffin tin greased with nonstick cooking spray or lined with paper cups. You should be able to get 6-8 jumbo

muffins or 15-16 regular sized muffins. Bake for 20 minutes or until the muffins are golden brown and the tops spring back when you press on them.

Notes

You can definitely get by with less sugar in this recipe by reducing the amount of maple syrup and honey. However, I liked the combination of both sweeteners together much better than either one of them on their own (for both taste and texture), so keep both if you can.

A.M. Snack (47 calories)

- 1/2 medium apple

Lunch (320 calories)

Green Salad with Spiced Chickpea "Nuts"

- 2 cups mixed greens
- 1/2 cup cucumber slices
- 5 cherry tomatoes, halved
- 1 Tbsp. feta cheese
- 5 Kalamata olives, pitted
    - 1/4 cup Spiced Chickpea "Nuts"

Combine ingredients and top salad with 1/2 Tbsp. each balsamic vinaigrette and olive oil.

P.M. Snack (51 calories)

- 6 dried apricots

Dinner (457 calories)

Roast Salmon with Fennel & Couscous

- 5 oz. roasted salmon fillet, coated with 1/4 tsp. olive oil, 1/4 teaspoon dried oregano and seasoned with a pinch each of salt and pepper
- 1 cup roasted fennel bulb, tossed with 1/2 Tbsp. olive oil and a pinch each of salt and pepper
- 1 cup cooked whole-wheat couscous topped with 1 Tbsp. chopped walnuts
- Lemon wedge as garnish

Evening Snack (37 calories)

- 1 medium fresh fig or 1 medium plum

Day 2:

Breakfast (297 calories)

1 Leftover zucchini muffin

A.M. Snack (70 calories)

- 2 clementines

Lunch (347 calories)

Mediterranean Tuna and antipasto salad
- ½ 15- to 19-ounce can beans, such as chickpeas, black-eyed peas or kidney beans, rinsed, or 1 7-ounce can
- 1 5- to 6-ounce can water-packed chunk light tuna, drained and flaked (see Note)
- ½ large red bell pepper, finely diced
- ¼ cup finely chopped red onion
- ¼ cup chopped fresh parsley, divided
- 2 teaspoons capers, rinsed
- ¾ teaspoon finely chopped fresh rosemary
- 4 tablespoons lemon juice, divided
- 2 tablespoons extra-virgin olive oil, divided
- Freshly ground pepper, to taste
- ⅛ teaspoon salt
- 4 cups mixed salad greens

1. Combine beans, tuna, bell pepper, onion, parsley, capers, rosemary, 2 tablespoons lemon juice and 1 tablespoon oil in a medium bowl. Season with pepper. Combine the remaining 2 tablespoons lemon juice, 1 tablespoon oil and salt in a large bowl. Add salad greens; toss to coat. Divide the greens between 2 plates. Top each with the tuna salad.

Note: Chunk light tuna, which comes from the smaller skipjack or yellowfin, has less mercury than canned white albacore tuna. The FDA/EPA advises that women who are or might become pregnant, nursing mothers and young children consume no more than 6 ounces of albacore a week; up to 12 ounces of canned light tuna is considered safe.

P.M. Snack (108 calories)

- 5 walnut halves
- 5 dried apricots

Dinner (427 calories)

- 1 3/4 cup Tomato and Artichoke Gnocchi
- 2 tablespoons extra-virgin olive oil, divided
- 1 16-ounce package shelf-stable gnocchi
- 1 small onion, sliced
- 1 small red bell pepper, diced
- 4 large cloves garlic, thinly sliced
- 1 tablespoon chopped fresh oregano, plus more for garnish
- 1 15-ounce can chickpeas, rinsed
- 1 14-ounce can no-salt-added diced tomatoes
- 1 9-ounce box frozen artichoke hearts, thawed and chopped
- 8 pitted Kalamata olives, sliced

- 1 tablespoon red-wine vinegar
- ¼ teaspoon ground pepper

Preparation

1. Heat 1 tablespoon oil in a large nonstick skillet over medium-high heat. Add gnocchi and cook, stirring often, until plumped and starting to brown, about 5 minutes. Transfer to a bowl and cover to keep warm.

2. Reduce heat to medium. Add the remaining 1 tablespoon oil and onion to the pan. Cook, stirring occasionally, until starting to brown, 2 to 3 minutes. Add bell pepper; cook, stirring occasionally, until crisp-tender, about 3 minutes. Add garlic and oregano; cook, stirring, for 30 seconds. Add chickpeas, tomatoes and artichokes; cook, stirring, until hot, about 3 minutes. Stir in olives, vinegar, pepper and the gnocchi. Sprinkle with oregano, if desired.

Day 3:

Breakfast (266 calories)

Egg & Toast Breakfast

- 1 slice whole-wheat bread, toasted
- 1/4 medium avocado, mashed
- 1 large egg, cooked in 1/4 tsp. olive oil or coat pan with a thin layer of cooking spray

(1-second spray). Season with a pinch each salt and pepper.

Top toast with mashed avocado and egg.

- 1 clementine

A.M. Snack (131 calories)

- 1/4 cup Spiced Chickpea "Nuts"

Lunch (332 calories)

Leftovers

- 1 cup Tomato & Artichoke Gnocchi
- 2 cups mixed greens

Top salad greens with 1/2 Tbsp. each balsamic vinaigrette & olive oil.

P.M. Snack (25 calories)

- 3 dried apricots

Dinner (314 calories)

Shiitake Mushroom Fettuccini With Basil

- 2 tablespoons extra-virgin olive oil
- 3 cloves garlic, minced
- 2 ounces shiitake mushrooms, stemmed and sliced (1½ cups)
- 2 teaspoons freshly grated lemon zest
- 2 tablespoons lemon juice, juice

- ¼ teaspoon salt, or to taste
- Freshly ground pepper, to taste
- 8 ounces whole-wheat fettuccine, or spaghetti (see Ingredient note)
- ½ cup chopped fresh basil, divided
- ½ cup freshly grated Parmesan cheese, (1 ounce)

1. Bring a large pot of lightly salted water to a boil for cooking pasta.
2. Heat oil in large nonstick skillet over low heat. Add garlic and cook, stirring, until fragrant but not browned, about 1 minute. Add mushrooms and increase heat to medium-high; cook, stirring occasionally, until tender and lightly browned, 4 to 5 minutes. Stir in lemon zest, lemon juice, salt and pepper. Remove from the heat.
3. Meanwhile, cook pasta, stirring occasionally, until just tender, 9 to 11 minutes or according to package directions. Drain, reserving ½ cup cooking liquid.
4. Add the pasta, the reserved cooking liquid, Parmesan and ¼ cup basil to the mushrooms in the skillet; toss to coat well. Serve immediately, garnished with remaining basil.
5. Ingredient Note: Whole-wheat pastas are higher in fiber than white pastas. They can

be found in health-food stores and some large supermarkets.

Day 4:

Breakfast (306 calories)

1 Cup Mediterranean Breakfast Couscous

- 3 cups 1% low-fat milk 1 (2-inch) cinnamon stick
- 1 cup uncooked whole-wheat couscous
- 1/2 cup chopped dried apricots
- 1/4 cup dried currants
- 6 teaspoons dark brown sugar, divided
- 1/4 teaspoon salt
- 4 teaspoons butter, melted and divided

1. Combine milk and cinnamon stick in a large saucepan over medium-high heat; heat 3 minutes or until small bubbles form around inner edge of pot (about 180°). Do not boil.
2. Remove from heat; stir in couscous, apricots, currants, 4 teaspoons brown sugar, and salt. Cover the mixture, and let it stand 15 minutes. Remove and discard cinnamon stick. Divide couscous among each of 4 bowls, and top each with 1 teaspoon melted butter and 1/2 teaspoon brown sugar. Serve immediately.

A.M. Snack (65 calories)

- 5 walnut halves

Lunch (350 calories)

Green Salad with Pita Bread & Hummus

- 2 cups mixed greens
- 1/2 cup sliced cucumber
- 2 Tbsp. grated carrot

Top salad with 1/2 Tbsp. each olive oil & balsamic vinegar

- Serve with 1 whole-wheat pita round (6-1/2-inch), toasted, with 3 Tbsp. hummus for dipping.

P.M. Snack (80 calories)

- 1/2 cup nonfat plain Greek yogurt topped with 1/4 cup sliced strawberries

Dinner (314 calories)

- 1 cup Left Over Shiitake Mushroom Fettuccine

Day 5:

Breakfast (297 calories)

Oatmeal with Fruit & Nuts

- 1/2 cup oatmeal cooked in 1/2 cup skim milk and 1/2 cup water
- 1/2 apple, diced
- 1 Tbsp. chopped walnuts

Top oatmeal with apple, walnuts and a pinch of cinnamon.

A.M. Snack (152 calories)

- 1/2 medium apple
- 1 Tbsp. peanut butter

Lunch (292 calories)

Classic Greek Salad

Ingredients

- 1 small red onion, halved and thinly sliced
- Kosher salt
- 1/4 cup red wine vinegar
- Grated zest and juice of 1 lemon
- 1 teaspoon honey
- 1 teaspoon dried oregano
- Freshly ground pepper
- 1/4 cup extra-virgin olive oil, plus more for drizzling
- 12 to 14 small vine-ripened tomatoes, quartered

- 1 cup kalamata olives, halved and pitted
- 5 Persian cucumbers
- 1 4-ounce block Greek feta cheese, packed in brine
- Fresh oregano leaves, for topping (optional)
- Soak the red onion in a bowl of heavily salted ice water, 15 minutes.

Meanwhile, whisk the vinegar, lemon zest and juice, honey, dried oregano, 1/2 teaspoon salt and 1/4 teaspoon pepper in a large bowl. Whisk in the olive oil in a slow, steady stream until emulsified. Add the tomatoes and olives and toss.

Peel the cucumbers, leaving alternating strips of green peel. Trim the ends, halve lengthwise and slice crosswise, about 1/2 inch thick; add to the bowl with the tomatoes. Drain the red onion, add to the bowl and toss.

Drain the feta and slice horizontally into 4 even rectangles. Divide the salad among plates. Top with the feta and oregano; drizzle with olive oil and season with pepper.

P.M. Snack (27 calories)

- 1/2 cup sliced strawberries

Dinner (400 calories)

- 1 serving Roast Pork, Asparagus & Cherry Tomato Bowl
- 2½ cups water plus 2 tablespoons, divided 1¼ cups bulgur
- ¾ teaspoon salt, divided
- 1 pound pork tenderloin, trimmed
- 1 teaspoon dried marjoram
- ¼ teaspoon ground pepper
- 2 tablespoons canola oil, divided
- 1 bunch asparagus, trimmed and cut into 1-inch pieces
- 1 large red onion, chopped
- 1 cup halved cherry tomatoes
- ½ cup finely chopped fresh parsley
- 2 teaspoons lemon zest
- 2 tablespoons lemon juice
- ¼ cup plain hummus

Preparation

1. Preheat oven to 400°F.
2. Bring 2½ cups water to a boil in a medium saucepan. Remove from heat and stir in bulgur and ¼ teaspoon salt. Cover and let stand until tender, about 20 minutes.
3. Meanwhile, sprinkle pork with marjoram, pepper and ¼ teaspoon salt. Heat 1

tablespoon oil in a large cast-iron or other ovenproof skillet over medium-high heat. Add the pork; cook, turning several times, until browned on all sides, 4 to 6 minutes.

4. Toss asparagus and onion with the remaining 1 tablespoon oil and ¼ teaspoon salt in a medium bowl. When the pork is browned, scatter the asparagus and onion around it. Transfer the pan to the oven and roast until an instant-read thermometer inserted in the center of the pork registers 145°F, 12 to 16 minutes. About 5 minutes before the pork is done, scatter the tomatoes over the vegetables in the pan.

5. Transfer the pork to a clean cutting board and let rest for 5 minutes before slicing. Toss the vegetables with the pan juices.

6. Drain any remaining liquid from the bulgur, then stir in parsley, lemon zest and lemon juice. Combine hummus and 2 tablespoons hot -water in a small bowl. Divide the bulgur among 4 bowls and top with the pork and vegetables; drizzle with the hummus sauce.

Evening Snack (37 calories)

- 1 medium fresh fig or 1 medium plum

Day 6:

Breakfast (279 calories)

- 1 slice whole-wheat toast
- 1 Tbsp. peanut butter
- 1 medium banana

A.M. Snack (78 calories)

- 1 hard-boiled egg seasoned with a pinch each of salt and pepper

Lunch (192 calories)

Mediterranean Stuffed Portabella Mushroom Caps

Ingredients

- 4 (4-inch) portobello caps (about 3/4 pound)
- 1/4 cup finely chopped onion
- 1/4 cup finely chopped celery
- 1/4 cup finely chopped carrot
- 1/4 cup finely chopped red bell pepper
- 1/4 cup finely chopped green bell pepper
- 1/4 teaspoon dried Italian seasoning
- 2 garlic cloves, minced
- Cooking spray
- 3 cups (1/4-inch) cubed French bread, toasted

- 1/2 cup vegetable broth
- 1/2 cup (2 ounces) feta cheese, crumbled
- 3 tablespoons low-fat balsamic vinaigrette, divided
- 4 teaspoons grated fresh Parmesan cheese
- 1/4 teaspoon black pepper
- 4 cups mixed salad greens

Preheat oven to 350°.

Remove stems from mushrooms, and finely chop stems to measure 1/4 cup. Discard remaining stems. Combine 1/4 cup chopped stems, onion, and next 6 ingredients (through garlic).

Heat a large nonstick skillet over medium heat; coat pan with cooking spray. Add onion mixture to pan; cook 10 minutes or until vegetables are tender. Combine onion mixture and bread in a large bowl, tossing to combine. Slowly add broth to bread mixture, tossing to coat. Add feta; toss gently.

Remove brown gills from the undersides of mushroom caps using a spoon; discard gills. Place mushrooms, stem side up, on a baking sheet coated with cooking spray. Brush mushrooms evenly with 1 tablespoon vinaigrette. Sprinkle Parmesan and black pepper evenly over mushrooms; top each with

1/2 cup bread mixture. Bake at 350° for 25 minutes or until mushrooms are tender.

Combine remaining 2 tablespoons vinaigrette and greens, tossing gently. Place 1 cup greens on each of 4 plates; top each serving with 1 mushroom.

P.M. Snack (95 calories)

- 1 medium apple

Dinner (444 calories)

- 1 serving Mediterranean Tuna Spinach Salad
- 1½ tablespoons tahini 1½ tablespoons lemon juice
- 1½ tablespoons water
- 1 5-ounce can chunk light tuna in water, drained
- 4 Kalamata olives, pitted and chopped
- 2 tablespoons feta cheese
- 2 tablespoons parsley
- 2 cups baby spinach
- 1 medium orange, peeled or sliced

Preparation

1. Whisk tahini, lemon juice and water together in a bowl. Add tuna, olives, feta and

parsley; stir to combine. Serve the tuna salad over 2 cups spinach, with the orange on the side.

- 1 slice whole-wheat bread, toasted.

Day 7:

Breakfast (266 calories)

Egg & Toast Breakfast

- 1 slice whole-wheat bread, toasted
- 1/4 medium avocado, mashed
- 1 large egg, cooked in 1/4 tsp. olive oil or coat pan with a thin layer of cooking spray (1-second spray). Season with a pinch each salt and pepper.

Top toast with mashed avocado and egg.

- 1 clementine

A.M. Snack (95 calories)

- 1 medium apple

Lunch (350 calories)

Green Salad with Pita Bread & Hummus

- 2 cups mixed greens
- 1/2 cup sliced cucumber
- 2 Tbsp. grated carrot

Top salad with 1/2 Tbsp. each olive oil & balsamic vinegar.

- Serve with 1 whole-wheat pita round (6-1/2-inch), toasted, with 3 Tbsp. hummus for dipping.

P.M. Snack (27 calories)

- 1/4 cup sliced strawberries

Dinner (400 calories)

Mediterranean Stuffed Tomatoes

- 2 large tomatoes 1/2 cup packaged garlic croutons
- 1/4 cup (1 ounce) crumbled goat cheese
- 1/4 cup sliced pitted kalamata olives
- 2 tablespoons reduced-fat vinaigrette or Italian salad dressing
- 2 tablespoons chopped fresh thyme or basil

1. Preheat broiler.
2. Cut tomatoes in half crosswise. Use your finger to push out and discard seeds; use a paring knife to cut out the pulp, leaving 2 shells. Chop pulp, and transfer to a medium bowl. Place hollowed tomatoes, cut sides down, on a paper towel; drain 5 minutes. Add croutons, goat cheese, olives, dressing, and thyme or basil to pulp; mix well. Mound mixture into hollowed tomatoes.

3. Place tomatoes on a baking sheet or broiler pan. Broil 4-5 inches from heat until hot and cheese melts (about 5 minutes). Serve immediately.

Shopping and Meal Prep Tips and Tricks

To make shopping easier, stock up on apples, dried fruit, figs, couscous, olive oil, oats, pita, whole wheat bread, and all the salad fixings at the beginning of the week.

A lot of these snacks can be prepared ahead of time such as hummus, roasted chickpeas, hard boiled eggs, tuna salad, and a good salad base. Meal planning will be easiest if you can manage to organize and prep at the beginning of your week. At the very least, if you know of some very busy days in your schedule, try to do as much of the prep work for dinner as possible ahead of time the day before. You can also pack lunches to go the day before.

To save money, make your own hummus and salad dressings from scratch at home. Making these yourself, you will also have more control of the ingredients and nutrition facts.

If you don't like a particular fruit for a snack or in your oatmeal, switch it out with something you do enjoy.

Most of these meals stick to roughly the same calorie count, so although this is a 7-day plan based on the consumption of 1,200 calories per day, you can switch some of these meals to other days of the week to get a taste you prefer.

Conclusion

It is my sincere hope that you might have liked all the recipes which have been mentioned in the book and once again thank you for getting this book and experimenting with the recipes.

About The Author

Davet Lebrun is born with the vision to promote *Mediterranean diet* among the masses. The author has written several research papers on the topic. He has served as an instructor promoting various cultural arts in University of San Francisco. He is currently living with his spouse in Texas.

www.ingramcontent.com/pod-product-compliance
Lightning Source LLC
LaVergne TN
LVHW011946070526
838202LV00054B/4815